Fever in Children

Padmasani Venkat Ramanan
Ramachandran Padmanabhan

Fever in Children

Case Based Learning

Springer

Padmasani Venkat Ramanan
Department of Pediatrics
Sri Ramachandra Institute of Higher Education and Research
Chennai, Tamil Nadu, India

Ramachandran Padmanabhan
Department of Pediatrics and Head-Division of Clinical Research
Sri Ramachandra Institute of Higher Education and Research
Chennai, Tamil Nadu, India

ISBN 978-981-97-9966-4 ISBN 978-981-97-9967-1 (eBook)
https://doi.org/10.1007/978-981-97-9967-1

This Springer imprint is published by the registered company Springer Nature Singapore Pte Ltd.
The registered company address is: 152 Beach Road, #21-01/04 Gateway East, Singapore 189721, Singapore

Preface

Fever is the most common reason for consultation with a pediatrician. In most cases, the cause is obvious and the treatment is straightforward; however, some cases can be challenging. Unfortunately, errors in managing fever in children are fairly common. These include leaving out vital questions while taking a history, missing clinical clues during the initial examination, failing to recognize the significance of some clinical and laboratory findings, and delaying the ordering of essential investigations. Between us, we have treated over 50,000 children with fever and have been training interns and postgraduates in treating fever for over three decades. Over the years, we have also made our share of mistakes. The lessons learnt are deeply embedded, and hopefully, we have not repeated them. We realized that our experience could be used to help others and thus decided to write this book for medical students and physicians who care for children.

In *Fever in Children*: *Case Based Learning*, we present 23 detailed case studies that illustrate a comprehensive approach to managing various presentations of fever in children. The causes of fever without a focus that are frequently overlooked in pediatric practice are presented, including infections, connective tissue diseases, malignancies, and other rare conditions. In each chapter, we have provided an abstract with the key message. We then present a case discussion in the format of a teaching ward round led by a professor. The case details are provided in a stepwise manner, and at each stage, there are questions with answers and explanations to describe the thought process of the treating physician until the final diagnosis is made. The discussion concludes with a brief word on the treatment and its outcome. We have listed the learning points at the end of each chapter to emphasize the take-home messages and to help the reader retain the practice points. Though the children we have discussed in this book belong to a particular region and certain causes of fever may be predominant in this region, we have tried to keep the differential diagnosis and discussions as broad-based and universal as possible.

The focus of this book is on the process of arriving at a diagnosis. Pathophysiology and treatment are not discussed in great detail, and readers are urged to refer to other resources for this. It is our hope that the readers will use these practical lessons to approach children with fever confidently and rationally.

We gratefully acknowledge the encouragement of our dear colleagues and the photos they contributed. We thank our patients—the children and their families—for trusting us to treat them and allowing us to share in the experience; our students who inspire us every day; and our families for their encouragement and support throughout the years.

We would also like to extend our gratitude to the Springer team. for their support and assistance in publishing this book.

Chennai, Tamil Nadu, India Ramachandran Padmanabhan
Chennai, Tamil Nadu, India Padmasani Venkat Ramanan

Competing Interests The authors declare that they have no competing financial or non-financial interests related to the content of this book.

About the Book

Fever in Children: Case Based learning presents the clinical details of 23 patients from the authors' experience, who presented with fever. These include some common causes of fever that are frequently overlooked in pediatric practice and some uncommon causes, including uncommon infections, connective tissue diseases, malignancies, and other rare conditions.

Each clinical vignette describes the history, physical examination, laboratory data, and course in the hospital. The format is unique as the narrative is in the form of a teaching ward round with faculty and residents; the differential diagnosis considered at each stage with explanations and process of confirming/ruling out the diagnosis is described systematically. Once the diagnosis is made, the etiopathogenesis, clinical features, and management of the condition are briefly described. The discussion concludes with a comment on the patient's outcome.

Relevant patient photographs, radiological images, laboratory data, and charts are incorporated into specific case studies. At the end of each case study, there are learning points and a brief bibliography.

We hope this book will prove useful for practicing pediatricians, those in training, and medical students.

Contents

1 Approach to a Child with Fever

Contents

1.1 Introduction

Fever is a common complaint with which parents come to the pediatrician's office. Though most previously healthy children in all age groups are more likely to have a benign, self-limited viral infection, the challenge is in identifying those with a serious bacterial infection (SBI) or any other condition that needs close monitoring or urgent intervention. The approach to a febrile child comprises a good medical history, a complete physical examination, and the judicious use of laboratory tests. Fever in children who are immunocompromised and nosocomial fever are not covered in this section.

In clinical practice, the approach to an immunocompetent febrile child depends on the duration of fever. For fever duration of less than 7 days, the approach is as follows.

1.2 History

It is important to ask what the body temperature was, and how it was recorded. Parents often interpret "warm to touch" and "head feels hot" as fever. Temperature recording is necessary for medical decision-making, such as recommending laboratory tests or starting empirical antibiotics. Parents should be asked to record the body

P. Venkat Ramanan, R. Padmanabhan, *Fever in Children*,
https://doi.org/10.1007/978-981-97-9967-1_1

temperature with a digital thermometer whenever fever is suspected. Traditional mercury thermometers are no longer recommended as there is a chance that the glass can break. The broken glass may injure the child, and there is a risk of environmental health hazard due to evaporated mercury. Commonly, a digital multiuse thermometer is used to measure temperature in the axilla at all ages. The tympanic membrane thermometers and temporal artery temperature measurements are inaccurate in children. Fever is indicated when thermometer readings are higher than the upper limit of normal-oral reading over 100 °F (37.8 °C) or armpit reading over 99 °F (37.2 °C). Less commonly used in clinical practice are the rectal or ear readings where a temperature over 100.4 °F (38 °C) indicates fever. Fever of ≥39 °C (102.2 °F) is always a matter of concern.

Inquiry about the environmental temperature is important. In summer, the hot weather can cause the body temperature to increase as babies sweat less, reducing their body's ability to cool down. Overwrapping can also cause the body temperature to increase. The mother can be asked to unwrap the infant and keep him/her in a cool room and recheck the body temperature.

System-specific symptoms may give a clue. Gastrointestinal infections cause vomiting, diarrhea, and abdominal pain; respiratory infections cause nasal stuffiness, sneezing, discharge, and cough; and urinary tract infection (UTI) may cause dysuria, increased frequency of micturition, and change in the color or odor of the urine. It is important to know when the child last passed urine to assess the adequacy of hydration.

Exposure to sick contacts in the household or daycare should be ascertained. Recent travel history is also important as it may give a clue to infections that are endemic in some regions.

History of previous illnesses and antibiotic use should be noted. Immunization history, especially for the vaccines not offered in the national immunization program, is important.

A family history of a previous death in a young infant from an infectious disease should alert one to the possibility of primary immune deficiencies.

1.3 Physical Examination

This includes the vital signs: temperature (38 °C = 100.4 °F), capillary refill time (CRT), pulse oximetry, and growth parameters with percentiles. A heart rate of more than 160 beats per minute in infants, a respiratory rate of more than 60 breaths per minute, and a prolonged CRT (=/> 3 s) often signal the development of septic shock. Irritability, inconsolability, cold extremities due to poor perfusion, poor tone, decreased activity, and lethargy can be signs of a serious infection. These children should be admitted for evaluation and empiric antibiotic therapy.

Clinical clues to specific infections should be identified by a thorough examination. Flushing (Fig. 1.1) is seen in dengue fever, skin rashes/mucous membrane enanthems are present in viral exanthematous illnesses, mucositis is seen in vasculitic disorders like Kawasaki disease (Fig. 1.2), periorbital edema due to third spacing is seen in dengue and scrub typhus, eschar particularly in the axillary folds, groin, gluteal clefts is pathognomonic of scrub typhus, and lymph node enlargement (Fig. 1.3) is seen in several conditions. Findings in extremities like joint or soft tissue swelling, warmth, redness, failure to bear weight, and pain on passive motion of an extremity should also be noted.

Foci of infection should be identified by ear examination for acute otitis media, throat examination for tonsillitis (Fig. 1.4), and examination of the systems.

Bacterial infections like urinary tract infections (UTIs), bacteremia, and pneumonia may not be clinically apparent on physical examination.

Following history and physical examination, fever is usually categorized as follows:

(a) Fever with localizing signs
(b) Fever without focus (FWF)

The management of fever with localizing signs will be fairly straightforward.

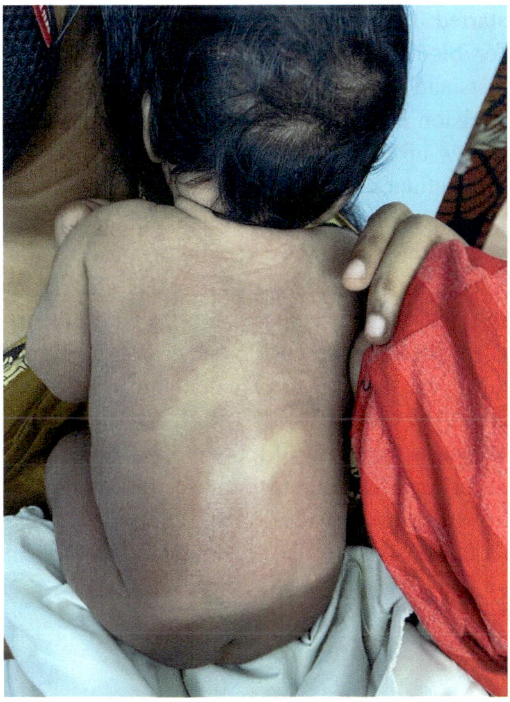

Fig. 1.1 Flushing in dengue fever with blanching in the areas of pressure with three fingers (Courtesy Dr. Dhanaratnamoorthy)

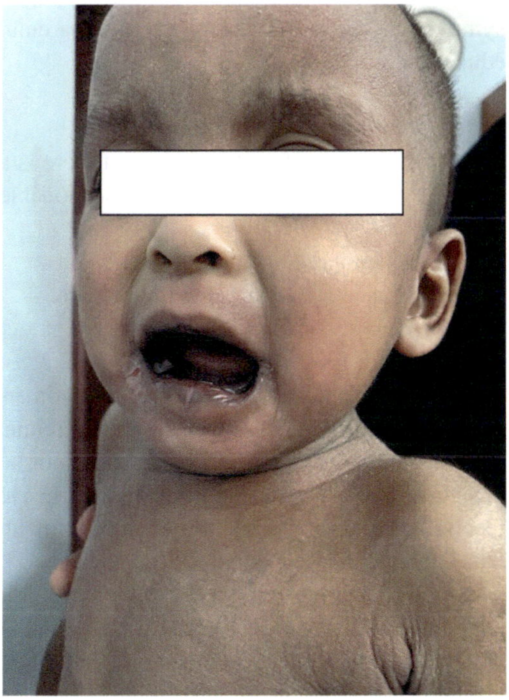

Fig. 1.2 Stomatitis in a child with Kawasaki disease (Courtesy Dr. Dhanaratnamoorthy)

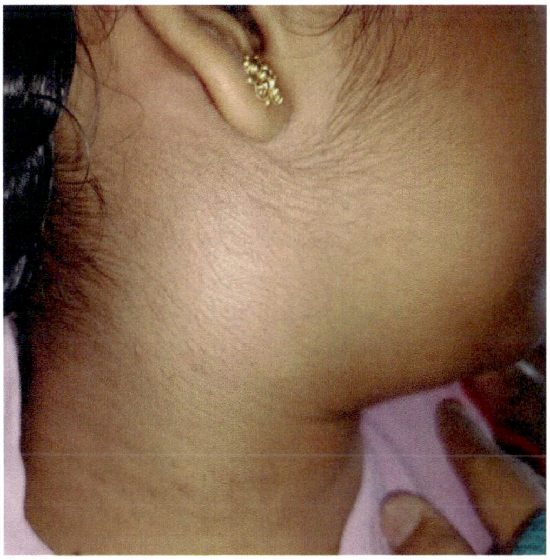

Fig. 1.3 Enlarged cervical lymph node (Courtesy Dr. S. Prasanna Kumar)

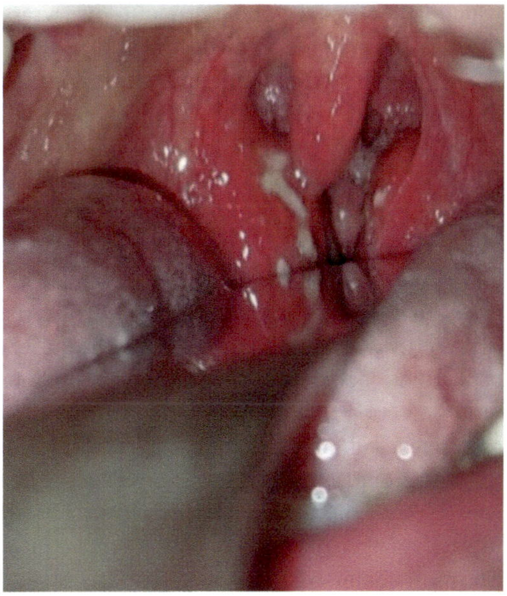

Fig. 1.4 Throat examination showing acute follicular tonsillitis (Courtesy Dr. S. Prasanna Kumar)

1.4 Fever Without Focus

Ill-appearing children and those with complex comorbidities or immunodeficiency are at a greater risk of serious bacterial infection (SBI). Such children should be hospitalized, investigated for sepsis, and given empiric antibiotic therapy.

In the assessment of well-appearing infants and young children, age and immunization status are important. The younger the infant, the greater is the concern as there are fewer clues on history and physical examination and a greater risk of a serious bacterial infection (SBI).

1.5 Neonates

All febrile neonates with documented fever, which is confirmed to be not due to overwrapping, should be hospitalized, investigated for sepsis, and started on empiric antibiotic therapy.

1.6 Infants 28 Days to <3 Months

SBI is seen in approximately 6–10%, and clinical evaluation alone is inadequate for identifying SBI in this age group. SBI may be present concurrently even in infants with an obvious viral infection. Bacterial meningitis is often associated with minimal signs and symptoms in this age group, and a bulging fontanelle is a late sign. Nuchal rigidity is only present in 27% of infants younger than 6 months with meningitis. The most common SBI is the urinary tract infection (UTI).

Currently There is No Consensus/Guidelines for Minimal Investigations to Be Done in a Febrile, Well-Appearing Infant. The author recommends a complete blood count (CBC), C reactive protein (CRP), and urine microscopy. If the infant has a WBC count of >15,000 cells/μL, absolute neutrophil count (ANC) of >10,000 cells/μL, or > 10 WBCs/HPF on urine microscopic examination, blood and urine culture should be done and empiric antibiotic should be started. To avoid multiple blood draws, a sample for blood culture is drawn with initial blood tests and held till the results are available. If the decision is made to not do blood tests, reliable follow-up is of utmost importance.

Usefulness of Acute Phase Reactants: Serum procalcitonin (PCT) is a useful test in settings where the results are rapidly available (turnaround time of 1 h or less). A value of >0.5 ng/mL has high specificity for bacterial illness. C-reactive protein (CRP) is superior to WBC and ANC, but inferior to procalcitonin in detecting SBI. At a threshold of 20 mg/L, C-reactive protein had a sensitivity of 100% (95% CI: 87–100%) and a negative predictive value of 100% (95% CI: 99–100%, prevalence of SBI: 2.8%).

1.7 Well-Appearing Child Aged 3 Months to 3 Years

Most well-appearing children with FWF have a self-limited viral illness. Immunization reactions may be a cause. Children with a low grade fever of <39 °C (102.2 F) can be managed symptomatically at home for 48 h with parental education on:

(a) Recognition of warning signs.
(b) Prophylaxis for febrile seizures (if there is a past history) though it is of questionable value.
(c) Paracetamol use and precautions.
(d) Importance of encouraging fluid intake.

Those with fever more than 39 °C (102.2 °F) are at risk of having a bacterial infection, primarily, urinary tract infections (UTIs), bacteremia, and pneumonia, and "viral fever" should not be presumed to be the cause. In children who have received the primary series of immunization with three doses of the conjugate vaccines against *S. pneumoniae* and type b *H. influenzae*, occult urinary tract infection (UTI) is the most common cause and urine routine examination and culture should be done. Samples collected by a urine bag are not useful. Urine for culture should be collected only by clean catch or catheterization. In areas endemic for dengue fever, dengue NS1 antigen and baseline CBC are useful in the first 4 days.

In unimmunized children, laboratory tests for CBC and CRP should be done and interpreted as given in the previous section. A chest radiograph is indicated in children with WBC >20,000/μL, even in the absence of respiratory symptoms. Though an infiltrate on radiograph cannot reliably identify whether a pneumonia is bacterial or viral, antibiotic treatment is indicated when there is leukocytosis. Tooth eruption should not be considered a source of fever.

1.8 Prolonged Fever

Fever of unknown origin (FUO) is defined as a temperature higher than 38 °C (100.4 °F) daily for at least 7–14 days (depending on whether it's a hospitalized or an outpatient) without a diagnosis on initial evaluation.

The common causes come under the following categories:

1. Infections: UTI/TB/osteomyelitis/brucellosis/scrub typhus/typhoid and infection associated with immune dysregulation.
2. Collagen vascular diseases.
3. Malignancies.
4. Miscellaneous.

The relative frequency of the individual conditions under these categories will vary depending on the age of the child, the geographic region, and the type of medical practice. In children, unusual presentations of common infections are the most common cause. The common infections identified include tuberculosis, enteric fever, urinary tract infection, osteomyelitis, and brucellosis. The evaluation of these children should proceed in a stepwise manner preferably after hospitalization. There is no standard algorithm for evaluating FUO. Diagnostic tests are best guided by ongoing assessment for historical, physical, and basic laboratory clues. Begin with the least invasive evaluation. This avoids unnecessary harm and cost to the patient. A "routine" battery of tests should be avoided as false leads will emerge. The tempo of the investigations will be determined by the clinical condition of the child. Hemodynamically unstable children or those with evidence of organ damage like hepatitis or myocarditis need rapid evaluation. Empiric antibiotics should never be started without collecting blood and urine cultures.

1.9 Parental Counseling on FWF

1. **What is the cause of my child's fever?**

   A: On clinical examination, the cause is not obvious. The typical causes in children are these, but in your child we cannot tell. We have to wait for the symptoms to evolve.
2. **Is it something serious?**

   A: At present the child is stable but in children we always need to be vigilant. You need to watch out for warning signs (Box 1.1) and report to the emergency room if any of them develops.
3. **He is refusing to take anything by mouth. What to do?**

   A: (If, in your assessment, child is active, hydration is good and vitals are normal) Children do refuse to eat during fever but try feeding during the inter-febrile period (after giving paracetamol). Keep offering liquids that are better accepted than solids. Watch for wet diaper and report if no urine has been passed for over 6 h. There are no medicines to "make the child eat." Patience and perseverance are the key. If intake is so poor that maintaining hydration is a concern, we will admit your child and maintain hydration with intravenous fluids.
4. **Can I give him paracetamol and send him to school? (Usually when both parents are working)**

   A: No. It is important for the child to stay at home with a responsible caretaker to encourage the child to eat and for rest and timely medication. Also, many illnesses are contagious.

Box 1.1 Parent Education on Warning Signs (Red Flags) in Children with Fever

- Inconsolable crying, irritability
- Difficulty in breathing
- Appearance of a rash
- Seizures
- Persistent vomiting
- Refusal to drink fluids
- Not passing urine for over 6 h
- Cold extremities
- Unusual tiredness
- A fever that reappears after dissipating for more than 24 h
- Fever that worsens or does not improve after 5 days

Learning Points

1. In the management of febrile children, the challenge is to identify those with a serious condition that needs urgent intervention or close monitoring.
2. All febrile neonates should be hospitalized, investigated for sepsis, and started on empiric antibiotic therapy.
3. Ill-appearing children and those with complex comorbidities or immunodeficiency are at a greater risk of SBI, regardless of their age.
4. For febrile children between 1 and 3 months of age, even if well-appearing, laboratory investigations to look for evidence of SBI are recommended. If the decision is made to not do blood tests, reliable follow-up is of utmost importance.
5. Well-appearing children, aged 3 months to 36 months, with fever <39 °C (102.2 °F) can be managed symptomatically with parental education on the red flags.
6. Those with fever >39 °C (102.2 °F) are at risk for bacterial infection, and occult urinary tract infection (UTI) is the most common cause in immunized children.
7. In areas endemic for dengue fever, dengue NS1 antigen and baseline CBC are useful in the first 4 days.
8. FUO for >7 days could be due to infectious or noninfectious causes.
9. In children, unusual presentations of common infections are the most common cause of FUO.
10. Evaluation of these children should proceed in a stepwise manner, preferably after hospitalization.

Suggested Readings

Burstein B, Alathari N, Papenburg J. Guideline-based risk stratification for febrile young infants without Procalcitonin measurement. Pediatrics. 2022;149:e2021056028.

Philbin D, Hall D. Fifteen-minute consultation: the approach to the febrile child. Arch Dis Child Educ Pract Ed. 2022;107(6):422–6. https://doi.org/10.1136/archdischild-2020-321335. Epub 2021 Aug 25.

Part I

Fever < 7 Days

2 Urinary Tract Infection

Contents

> **Key Messages**
> Fever may be the only manifestation of UTI in young children, and a febrile UTI may be the first manifestation of an anatomical abnormality of the urinary tract.

2.1 Case Discussion

A 9-month-old boy presented to the emergency room at 11.30 pm with an abrupt onset of fever documented to be 103.4 F in the axilla by the emergency room staff. With oral paracetamol, the child's fever subsided and the child was otherwise playful and active. On history, there were no localizing respiratory, gastrointestinal, or urinary symptoms. The child was fully immunized according to the national immunization program, with the last vaccine taken being the MR vaccine at 9 months 2 weeks earlier. On examination, the vital signs were normal and the anterior fontanel was flat. There were no clinical findings to suggest a focus of infection.

Since the fever had come down and the child was playful, the parents wished to go home.

1. *What is your diagnosis and what would you advise the parents?*

This child has a fever without focus, and a label of "viral fever" should not be given to such children. As the child is well-appearing and hemodynamically stable, hospitalization is not indicated. However, a fever of more than 39 °C (102.2 F) may indicate a bacterial infection. In children who have received the primary series of immunizations with conjugate vaccines against *Streptococcus pneumoniae* and *Haemophilus Influenzae* type b, occult urinary tract infection (UTI) is the most commonly occurring bacterial infection. In young children, urinary symptoms may not be present, and fever may be the only manifestation of UTI. Hence, urine routine and

P. Venkat Ramanan, R. Padmanabhan, *Fever in Children*,
https://doi.org/10.1007/978-981-97-9967-1_2

culture should be sent, and the child should be reviewed with the report.

2. *What are the specific points to be noted on physical examination in a child with suspected UTI?*

Physical examination in a child with suspected UTI should include:

(a) Blood pressure measurement: Acute pyelonephritis may cause renal scarring, and elevated blood pressure may indicate renal scarring.
(b) Abdominal palpation: Suprapubic and renal angle tenderness may be present in cystitis and pyelonephritis, respectively. A palpable bladder or kidney may indicate urinary obstruction. A palpable loaded colon may indicate constipation, a risk factor for UTI.
(c) Examination of the external genitalia for phimosis (Fig. 2.1), hypospadias, or labial adhesions.
(d) Examination of the lower back for signs of occult spina bifida.

In this child urine routine examination and culture were advised. The child has not passed urine for over an hour in the ER and the parents wanted to go back home, collect urine whenever he passed urine next, and bring the urine sample to the laboratory the next morning.

3. *What would be the ideal way to collect a urine sample when UTI is suspected?*

In infants and young children, the urine sample is preferably collected by catheterization or suprapubic aspiration for culture. A sample collected by urine bag is not useful for culture but can be used for dipstick and microscopy as a first step to determine whether a catheterized urine sample should be obtained. In children who are toilet trained, a mid-stream clean-voided specimen is preferred.

All urine specimens should be examined as soon as possible after collection and processed for culture within 30 min. Hence, parents should be urged to provide the sample before going home. In case of difficulty in culturing within 4 h of collection, urine can be refrigerated and transported within 24 h. If the sample is stored for even a few hours at room temperature both the false-positive and false-negative rates increase.

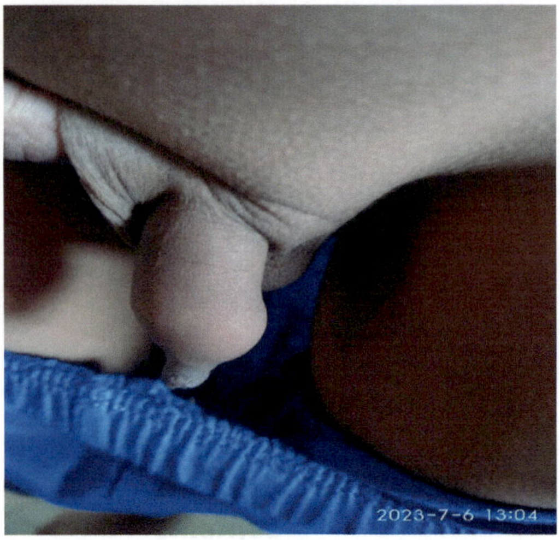

Fig. 2.1 Tight phimosis (Courtesy Dr. P. Ramachandran)

Table 2.1 Urine analysis report

Parameter	Report
Urine automated photometry	pH 7.0
Glucose, protein, ketones, urobilinogen	Negative
Nitrites	Positive
Leukocyte esterase	+++
Urine automated microscopy	Pus cells 18–20/HPF (ref interval < 5/HPF)

In this child, urine sample was collected by catheterization, and the urine analysis report is given in Table 2.1.

4. *How long does it take to get a urine analysis report and what features in the report would suggest the diagnosis of UTI?*

The reports of dipstick analysis and urine microscopy are usually available within 60 min in most laboratories. Dipsticks are reagent strips that are introduced to the urine sample. Color changes are read manually using the color chart on the container. Urine culture would take 48–72 h.

(a) Dipstick: A positive leukocyte esterase on dipstick analysis is suggestive of UTI but white blood cells (WBCs) may be present in the urine in other conditions as well—such as in acute appendicitis, group A streptococcal infection, and Kawasaki disease. Positive nitrite test on dipstick analysis is highly specific for UTI. It has a low false-positive rate, but false-negative rate is high as urine must remain in the bladder for at least 4 h for a detectable amount of nitrite. This is especially a problem in young infants who void more frequently.

(b) Microscopic examination: In standard microscopy, a centrifuged sample of unstained urine is examined for WBCs and bacteria. Pyuria is defined as ≥5 WBCs/high-power field (HPF), and bacteriuria as any bacteria per HPF. Enhanced microscopy is the examination of an uncentrifuged urine specimen using a hemocytometer and a Gram-stained smear. Here, pyuria is defined as ≥10 WBC/mm^3, and bacteriuria as any bacteria per 10 oil immersion fields of a Gram-stained smear. Automated microscopy uses flow cytometry and microscopic analyzers to detect WBC and bacteria. The definitions of pyuria and bacteriuria vary with the automated system. Urinary tract infection may be present without pyuria and most cases of bacteriuria without pyuria are observed in children with colonization due to *E. coli.*

(c) Urine culture: The definition of UTI is a significant bacteriuria of a clinically relevant uropathogen. Significant bacteriuria in a clean-voided sample is ≥100,000 colony-forming units (CFU)/mL of a single uropathogen, and for a catheter sample, it is ≥10,000 (10^4) CFU/mL.

5. *Is it important to send blood tests as well?*

Blood tests are not particularly helpful in diagnosing UTI and are not routinely necessary. Markers of inflammation like erythrocyte sedimentation rate (ESR), C-reactive protein (CRP), or procalcitonin (PCT) do not reliably differentiate between cystitis and pyelonephritis. When available, CRP <20 mg/L (2 mg/dL) makes pyelonephritis less likely and PCT >0.5 ng/mL (0.5 mcg/L) suggests pyelonephritis. Measurement of serum creatinine is not routinely necessary but is essential when there is a history of multiple UTI or if acute kidney injury due to dehydration or sepsis is suspected. Blood culture is not needed as a positive blood culture rarely alters management because the same organism usually is isolated from the blood and urine.

6. *Should antibiotics be started empirically in children with suspected UTI or only when confirmed by the urine culture reports?*

Early antibiotic therapy (within 72 h of presentation) may prevent kidney damage. Empiric antimicrobial therapy is important for children with suspected kidney involvement as they are at increased risk for kidney scarring. This includes ill-appearing children and those with fever ≥39 °C [102.2 °F] or for >48 h, renal angle tenderness, and known immune deficiency or urologic abnormality (e.g., Grade IV or V vesicoureteral reflux). It is important to collect urine appropriately for culture and antibiotic sensitivity before initiating empiric therapy.

7. *Do children with UTI need hospitalization?*

Children older than 3 months with UTI who are not vomiting can be safely managed as outpatients as long as close follow-up is possible; the seriousness of the infection and the need for the completion of the entire course of therapy should be emphasized. Hospitalization and parenteral therapy are indicated for age < 2 months, urosepsis (toxic appearance, hypotension, poor capillary refill), those with vomiting or inability to tolerate the oral medication, and when the response to outpatient therapy is inadequate.

8. *What is the antibiotic of choice for empiric therapy?*

The antibiotic of choice should be guided by local resistance patterns. The most common bacterial cause of UTI in infants and children is *E. coli* (>70%), and in most communities, they are resistant to amoxicillin, amoxicillin–clavulanate, and trimethoprim–sulfamethoxazole (TMP-SMX). Empiric treatment is started with a third-generation cephalosporin (oral cefixime 10 mg/kg daily in two divided doses), parenteral cefotaxime (150 mg/kg per day IV divided in three doses), or ceftriaxone (50–75 mg/kg per day IV; maximum daily dose 2 g) or an aminoglycoside. When the local resistance of *E. coli* to third-generation cephalosporins is high (ESBL producing organisms), one of the second-line antibiotics such as piperacillin–tazobactam should be chosen.

This child was started on oral cefixime after seeing the urine routine report which was highly suggestive of UTI. The parents came back after 3 days to the outpatient clinic with the culture reports. The child was afebrile. The culture report is detailed in Table 2.2.

9. *Should the antibiotic be changed now? What is the treatment duration? Should urine culture be repeated at any point?*

Once culture results become available, if the pathogen is resistant to empiric therapy, some experts would not change therapy if the child is clinically improving, while others would change the antibiotic to one to which the pathogen is sensitive. In this child, the same antibiotic was continued.

The treatment course is usually 10 days in uncomplicated UTI. Oral antibiotics can be used to complete the course of therapy for patients in whom treatment was initiated with parenteral antibiotics. Once the patient clinically improves, tolerates oral fluids, and has been afebrile for 24 h, we generally switch to oral antibiotics. Repeat urine culture is not needed in children who are treated with an antibiotic to which their uropathogen is susceptible.

Table 2.2 Urine culture report

Organism isolated: *Escherichia coli* > 10,000 CFU/mL	
Antibiotic	Susceptibility
Amikacin	Susceptible
Ampicillin	Resistant
Cefoperazone with sulbactam	Susceptible
Cefuroxime	Resistant
Cefotaxime	Resistant
Cotrimoxazole	Resistant
Nitrofurantoin	Susceptible
Norfloxacin	Resistant
Piperacillin tazobactam	Susceptible

10. *How soon does a child typically respond?*

The clinical condition usually improves within 48 h of initiation of appropriate antimicrobial therapy. If there is no improvement, the addition of ampicillin or amoxicillin may be warranted as most of the empiric regimens do not cover *Enterococcus*. Also, an ultrasonography (USG) should be performed to evaluate for a renal abscess.

11. *What is the current recommendation for imaging in young children with UTI?*

About 10% of children presenting with a single UTI and 50% of children with recurrent UTI have an associated urological abnormality. The rationale for imaging in young children with UTI is to identify abnormalities (e.g., obstructive uropathies, vesicoureteral reflux [VUR]) that require additional management to prevent UTI recurrence and kidney damage.

Ultrasonography: USG of the kidneys, ureters, and bladder (USG KUB) can demonstrate the size and shape of the kidneys, anatomic abnormalities like a posterior urethral valve, duplication and dilatation of the ureters, and renal and perirenal abscess or pyonephrosis. The Indian Academy of Pediatrics (IAP) recommends USG KUB in all children with UTI. The American Academy of Pediatrics (AAP) recommends USG for all infants and children 2–24 months following their first febrile UTI. The United Kingdom's National Institute for Health and Care Excellence (NICE) guidelines recommend ultrasonography for infants younger than 6 months and for children older than 6 months who have atypical or recurrent UTI. Atypical UTI is defined as serious illness, poor urine flow, abdominal or bladder mass, elevated creatinine, septicemia, infection with an organism other than *E. coli*, and failure to respond to antibiotics within 48 h; recurrence is defined as ≥2 episodes of upper UTI, 1 episode of upper UTI plus ≥1 episode of lower UTI, or ≥ 3 episodes of lower UTI.

Timing: In infants and young children with unusually severe illness or failure to improve as expected after initiation of antimicrobial therapy, USG should be performed during the acute phase of illness to identify complications (e.g., kidney or perirenal abscess, pyonephrosis). In those who respond as expected, USG should be performed after the acute phase (to reduce the risk of false-positive results secondary to kidney inflammation during the acute episode).

Micturating Cystourethrogram (MCU)—An MCU Is done to detect VUR (Fig. 2.2)

VUR is an important risk factor for kidney scarring. Approximately 25–30% of children (0–18 years) with a first UTI have VUR. The IAP recommends MCU in all children with UTI aged <1 year, and for older children, if DMSA is abnormal.

The AAP recommends postponing MCU until the second febrile UTI in children 2–24 months of age unless there are atypical or complex clinical circumstances or the USG reveals abnormalities suggestive of high-grade (IV or V) VUR or obstructive uropathy.

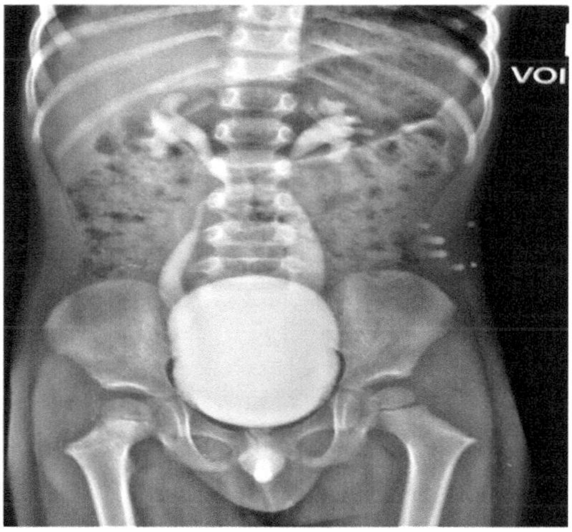

Fig. 2.2 Micturating cystourethrogram (MCU) showing Grade IV vesicoureteral reflux (VUR). (Courtesy Dr. Sangeetha Perungo)

The NICE guidelines suggest MCU for infants <6 months with atypical or recurrent UTI and for children 6 months to 3 years with atypical or recurrent UTI and dilation on ultrasonography, poor urine flow, non-*E. coli* infection, or family history of VUR.

Timing: Early imaging (as early as the first week) does not appear to falsely increase the detection of VUR. To avoid the use of prophylactic antibiotics in children without VUR, MCU is best done immediately after completion of antimicrobial therapy for UTI.

Dimercaptosuccinic acid [DMSA] scan: DMSA scan using technetium Tc-99m succimer can detect kidney scarring. The AAP and NICE guidelines do not recommend DMSA in the routine evaluation of children with first UTI. The NICE guidelines recommend DMSA 4–6 months after acute infection for children younger than 3 years with atypical or recurrent UTI and for children older than 3 years with recurrent UTI. The IAP recommendations for children with UTI are as follows:

1. Age < 1 year: USG and MCU, DMSA after 4–6 months.
2. Age 1–5 years: USG, DMSA after 4–6 months. MCU if DMSA is abnormal.
3. Age > 5 years: USG. DMSA and MCU only if USG is abnormal.

12. *What are the other important aspects of management after the first episode of UTI?*

Parents should be instructed to seek prompt evaluation for subsequent febrile illnesses to ensure prompt recognition and treatment of recurrent UTI. The evaluation of these episodes should include urinalysis and urine culture.

Identification and treatment of bowel and bladder dysfunction that predisposes many children to UTI may be more important than identifying anatomic or functional genitourinary abnormalities after the first febrile UTI in preventing recurrent UTI and kidney scarring.

2.2 Conclusion

The child was found to have a posterior urethral valve on USG and MCU. He underwent fulguration, after which he remained asymptomatic on follow-up.

Learning Points

1. In children younger than 2 years, urinary symptoms may not be present and fever may be the only manifestation of UTI.
2. Empiric antimicrobial therapy is important for children with suspected kidney involvement.
3. Early antibiotic therapy (within 72 h of presentation) may prevent kidney damage.
4. Urine sample should be collected before starting antibiotics for routine analysis and culture, in infants and young children by catheterization or suprapubic aspiration. The sample collected by urine bag is not useful.
5. *E. coli* is the most common pathogen causing UTI. The antibiotic of choice should be guided by local resistance patterns.
6. About 10% of children presenting with a single UTI and 50% of children with recurrent UTI have an associated urological abnormality. Hence, imaging is necessary according to the guidelines.
7. Identification and treatment of bowel and bladder dysfunction that predisposes many children to UTI is important.

Suggested Readings

‘t Hoen LA, Bogaert G, Radmayr C, Dogan HS, Nijman RJM, Quaedackers J, Rawashdeh YF, Silay MS, Tekgul S, Bhatt NR, Stein R. Update of the EAU/ESPU guidelines on urinary tract infections in children. J Pediatr Urol. 2021;17(2):200–7. https://doi.org/10.1016/j.jpurol.2021.01.037. Epub 2021 Feb 2. Erratum in: J Pediatr Urol. 2021 Aug;17(4):598.

Indian Academy of Pediatrics Standard Treatment Guideline. 2022. Urinary Tract Infection in children. https://iapindia.org/pdf/STG-06-Urinary-Tract-Infection-in-Children.pdf.

Mattoo TK, Shaikh N, Nelson CP. Contemporary management of urinary tract infection in children. Pediatrics. 2021;147(2):e2020012138.

3 Pneumonia

Contents

> **Key Messages**
> Pneumonia can present as fever without focus and without cough in young infants. A clinical diagnosis of pneumonia can be made in a child with fever and rapid/difficult breathing even without auscultation or a chest X-ray.

3.1 Case Discussion

A two-year-old girl, developmentally normal, was brought with a history of high-grade fever for 2 days without any localizing signs. She was not taking feeds well and had vomited a few times. Her sleep was disturbed, and she was not as active as usual. There was no history suggestive of foreign body aspiration or wheeze. There were no significant illnesses, hospitalization, or wheezing episodes in the past. She was the first child for the parents, and both parents were in good health. Her birth history was normal. She had been immunized with all the vaccines as per the national immunization schedule. Last vaccines were given at 17 months of age. There was no exposure to smoke or any indoor or outdoor air pollutant. There was no contact history of tuberculosis.

On examination, the child appeared ill and irritable. There was no pallor, duskiness, palpable lymph nodes, or pedal edema. She appeared to be dehydrated. She had a temperature of 101 °F, pulse rate of 124 per minute, respiratory rate of 72 per minute, and BP of 90/64 mmHg, and her peripheral pulses were well felt. Oxygen saturation was 92% in room air which improved to 98% with supplemental oxygen. She had lower chest wall indrawing and flaring of alae nasi. There was no audible sound such as stridor, wheeze, or grunt. Auscultation of the respiratory system was difficult in the ER in view of the child's restlessness. The cardiovascular system was normal. Abdominal examination revealed a soft and nontender liver of 2 cm below right costal margin, and the liver span was 6 cm which was normal. There were no signs of meningeal irritation. A clinical diagnosis of pneumonia was made.

P. Venkat Ramanan, R. Padmanabhan, *Fever in Children*,
https://doi.org/10.1007/978-981-97-9967-1_3

1. *What is pneumonia and what are the common presentations of respiratory infection in children?*

Respiratory infections are a common cause of fever, especially in young children. They are broadly divided into upper respiratory tract infections (URTIs) and lower respiratory tract infections (LRTIs). Upper respiratory infections causing significant fever are rhinitis, pharyngotonsillitis, sinusitis, and otitis media. Lower respiratory infections include tracheitis, bronchitis, bronchiolitis, pneumonia, and pleural infections. Among these, bronchiolitis and pneumonia are the major contributors to under 5 mortality, morbidity, and hospitalization.

Pneumonia indicates alveolar inflammation, and it can be community-acquired or hospital-acquired (nosocomial). Pneumonia contributes to around 13.5% of deaths in children aged 1–59 months and 7% of deaths in children aged 5–9 years.

2. *How is pneumonia diagnosed?*

A clinical diagnosis of pneumonia is made when the classical features of fever, cough, fast breathing, and difficult breathing are present. Cough may not be a predominant symptom in the initial phase, and auscultation in young children is difficult. Fever may be of varying degrees, and in young infants with pneumonia with certain organisms like *Chlamydia trachomatis*, fever may be absent (afebrile pneumonia). Conversely, fever may be the only manifestation of pneumonia in young children especially when associated with a high white blood cell count. Neonates and young infants with pneumonia may present with fever, irritability, inability to sleep, and feeding difficulty rather than cough. Older children may present with unilateral chest pain due to pleural inflammation or abdominal pain due to referred pain from the irritation of the diaphragmatic pleura. On examination of the chest, the presence of crackles, bronchial breathing, and impaired percussion note in a localized area of lung favor the diagnosis of pneumonia. Among the clinical signs, chest retraction and hypoxia (<94% in room air) are more predictive of pneumonia.

The World Health Organization (WHO) guidelines state that in children under 5 years of age who have cough, with or without fever, pneumonia is diagnosed by the presence of either fast breathing (tachypnea) or lower chest wall indrawing. Though fast breathing is a simple clinical sign with a high sensitivity, there are certain caveats. The respiratory rate (RR) should be counted for one full minute in a quiet child. The clinician would do well to be opportunistic and count the abdominal movement which is easier to visualize without even fully undressing and disturbing the child. The WHO has given guidelines on age-specific cutoff for the respiratory rate to define fast breathing. These are:

1. <2mo: ≥60/min
2. 2 mo to <12 mo: ≥50/min
3. 12 mo to 59 mo: ≥40/min
4. ≥5 years: ≥20/min.

Other causes of tachypnea (viral associated wheeze, asthma, congestive heart failure, metabolic acidosis) should be considered in the appropriate clinical context. Increased work of breathing may involve intercostal, subcostal, suprasternal, and sternal retractions, grunting, and nasal flaring. The WHO has emphasized on lower chest wall indrawing as the more specific characteristic of pneumonia in young infants.

General examination of a child suspected to have pneumonia should focus on the assessment of airway, breathing, and circulation including oxygen saturation by pulse oximetry. Any altered level of consciousness, severe chest indrawing, cyanosis, apnea, or features of shock require immediate intervention to stabilize the child.

The child was admitted with a diagnosis of severe pneumonia and respiratory distress with impending respiratory failure. She was started on oxygen by face mask which she tolerated well, and the saturation improved to 98%. Intravenous (IV) fluids were required for the first 24 h of hospitalization as she was dehydrated, and there was respiratory distress. IV ceftriaxone was started. Her chest X-ray (CXR) revealed left upper lobe opacity with air bronchogram (Fig. 3.1).

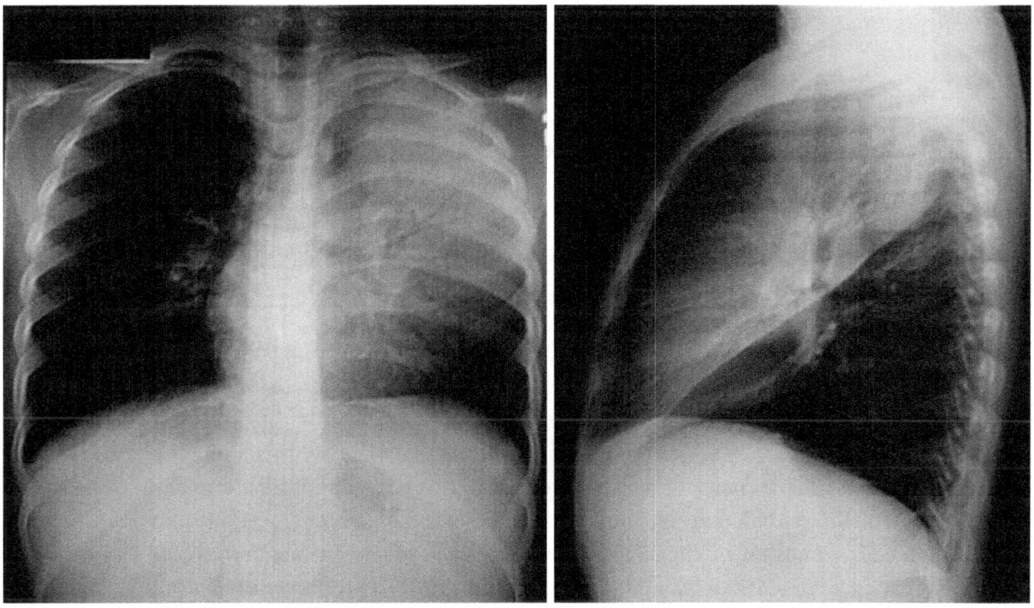

Fig. 3.1 CXR: Pneumonia left upper lobe

3. *How is the severity of pneumonia assessed?*

The WHO has categorized the severity in children aged 2–59 months as "pneumonia" and "severe pneumonia." In a child with cough and/or difficult breathing, "fast breathing and/or chest indrawing" suggest "pneumonia," and the presence of general danger signs (not able to drink, persistent vomiting, convulsions, lethargy or unconsciousness, stridor in a calm child, or severe malnutrition) suggests "severe pneumonia." This classification is helpful in deciding the type of management and the facility in which the child should be managed.

In clinical practice, age less than 3 months, severe pneumonia, underlying medical conditions, disadvantaged socioeconomic status, and failure of outpatient treatment are considered indicators for inpatient care. Physiologic status of respiration is classified as respiratory distress or respiratory failure as per the Pediatric Advanced Life Support (PALS) guidelines. This approach helps decide the rapidity and level of immediate intervention.

4. *What are the causative organisms of pneumonia?*

Community-acquired pneumonia (CAP) can be caused by both viruses and bacteria. It can also be mixed infection (viral and bacterial). The etiology of pneumonia is dynamic due to the use of vaccines. With widespread uptake of Hib vaccine and PCV, viruses are the predominant cause of pneumonia, but bacteria continue to cause from a quarter to a third of all cases. According to the WHO report (Pneumonia in children 2022), *Streptococcus pneumoniae* (*S. pneumoniae*) is the most common cause of bacterial CAP in children followed by *Hemophilus influenzae* type b (Hib). Respiratory syncytial virus (RSV) is the most common viral cause of pneumonia. The other viruses implicated are human metapneumovirus (hMPV), rhinovirus, parainfluenza virus 1, 3, and 4, and influenza virus A and B. Atypical organisms such as *Mycoplasma pneumoniae* (*M. pneumoniae*) are more commonly seen in school-age children (after 5 years of age). Unusual organisms may be associated with pneumonia in children with underlying conditions such as immunodeficiency or cystic fibrosis. In newborns and young infants <3 mo of age, gram-negative bacilli, *C. trachomatis*, viruses, and *S. pneumoniae* are the predominant causative organisms. In infants infected with HIV, *Pneumocystis jirovecii* is one of the most common causes of pneumonia.

5. *Are there any clues for etiology in the clinical examination?*

Wheezing is commonly associated with viral infections and atypical organisms such as *M. pneumoniae*. The presence of extrapulmonary manifestations such as myalgia, arthralgia, mucocutaneous lesions of various types, hemolytic anemia, pancreatitis, hepatitis, and myocarditis may point toward a diagnosis of *M. pneumoniae*. Young age (1–4 mo) and associated conjunctivitis may indicate infection due to *Chlamydia trachomatis*, *Mycoplasma hominis*, and *Ureaplasma urealyticum*. Clinical features of pneumonia due to bacterial, viral, and atypical organisms frequently overlap. Stony dull note on percussion and absent breath sounds may indicate the development of a complication like pleural effusion which frequently occurs with *Staphylococcus aureus or Streptococcus pneumoniae*.

6. *What is the role of CXR and other imaging modalities in a child suspected to have pneumonia?*

Chest X-ray (CXR) is not necessary in children managed as outpatients. It is usually taken in all children admitted for pneumonia. In young children 3–36 months of age presenting with fever without focus and a high total leukocyte count of >20,000/cmm, a CXR may be required to rule out occult pneumonia. It should be emphasized that the CXR features will not reliably differentiate bacterial, viral, or mycoplasma infections as there is considerable overlap. There may be a few useful clues for bacterial pneumonia in CXR such as (1) lobar consolidation, (2) a "round" pneumonia (commonly due to *S. pneumoniae*, sometimes, *S. aureus*, *Klebsiella*), (3) pneumatoceles, and necrotizing pneumonia. Lung ultrasonography (LUS) is shown to be a good modality to identify pneumonia, and its scope has increased tremendously with improved operator expertise and technology. LUS is useful to follow the progression and/or resolution of CAP. Computed tomographic scan (CT scan) of the chest may be required in a sick child with unresolving pneumonia to identify complications such as necrotizing pneumonia or lung abscess, but it should be used judiciously in view of the risk of exposure to ionizing radiation. LUS is applied increasingly more to identify even these complications.

7. *What are the other investigations required in a child with pneumonia?*

Children with CAP treated with ambulatory care do not require any investigation. Hospitalized children, in view of the severity of the condition, require complete work-up for infection. The total leukocyte count will generally be >15,000/cmm in bacterial pneumonia but can be raised in adenovirus and *M.* pneumoniae pneumonia also. Acute phase reactants such as erythrocyte sedimentation rate (ESR), C-reactive protein (CRP), and serum procalcitonin (PCT), though raised in pneumonia, are not specific for bacterial pneumonia. On the other hand, serial CRP and PCT are useful to monitor the clinical response to therapy in pneumonia. Normal CRP and PCT values help in ruling out a bacterial etiology. Blood cultures are indicated in hospitalized children. Though the yield is <10%, it is useful to attempt to identify the etiology in view of the serious nature of the disease. *S. pneumoniae* is the leading bacterial organism identified in blood culture followed by *S. aureus* and *S. pyogenes*. Ancillary investigations such as serum electrolytes, liver function test, and renal function test may be required in critically ill children requiring intensive care. They may also require arterial blood gases in preparation for and during ventilation therapy.

Laboratory reports are as follows: hemoglobin 10.8 g/dL (Normal 11.5–14.5 g/dL); total leukocyte count (TLC) 18,400/cmm (4000–12,000/cmm), differential leucocyte count (DLC) showed neutrophils 80% (54–62%), lymphocytes 16% (25–33%), eosinophils 1% (1–3%), monocytes 2.6% (3–7%), and basophils 0.4% (0–0.75%); platelet count 340,000/cmm (150,000–400,000/cmm). C-reactive protein was 9.2 mg/dL (normal <0.6 mg/dL). Serum electrolyte estimation revealed sodium, potassium, and chloride levels to be 128mMol/L, 4.2mMol/L, and 92mMol/L, respectively. Blood culture was sterile.

8. *What is the role of rapid diagnostic tests in pneumonia?*

These are polymerase chain reaction (PCR)-based molecular tests done in nasopharyngeal, throat, or pleural fluid samples. Multiplex PCR panels are used to test common respiratory viruses and bacteria simultaneously. It must be remembered that the organisms identified from the upper respiratory tract (URT) may be just the resident organisms at that site and cannot be confirmed to be responsible for the LRTI. The causal association with LRTI is seen more with RSV, influenza virus, parainfluenza virus, and hMPV identified from URT. Identification of RSV may aid in cohorting the patients in the hospital. Antiviral therapy can be started in severe respiratory infection when influenza virus is identified. In suspected *M. pneumoniae* infection, PCR test from throat swab is very useful.

9. *What are the predisposing factors for severity of pneumonia?*

The identified risk factors for childhood pneumonia are undernutrition, incomplete immunization, indoor pollution due to the use of solid fuels in the household, lack of exclusive breastfeeding, low maternal educational status, and limited access to health care. In a multi-centric study over five centers in India, younger age and undernutrition were the identifiable risk factors for both CAP and severe CAP.

10. *How is pneumonia treated?*

The choice of treatment is based on age, the likely pathogen, and any underlying host factors.

- Children less than 3 months of age with CAP are treated as inpatients with parenteral antibiotics irrespective of the severity.
- For outpatient treatment of pneumonia, oral antibiotics are used.
  - Age: 3–59 months: amoxicillin 80 mg/kg/day × 5 days; co-amoxiclav as second line.
  - Age: 5 years or more: amoxicillin as above; co-amoxiclav/azithromycin as second line
- For inpatient treatment, parenteral antibiotics are used.
  - Age < 3 months: cefotaxime or ceftriaxone; piperacillin-tazobactam with or without gentamycin/amikacin as second line.
  - Age 3–59 months: ampicillin; co-amoxiclav/cefotaxime/ceftriaxone as second line.
  - Age ≥ 5 years: ampicillin; co-amoxiclav/cefotaxime/ceftriaxone/azithromycin as second line.
  - In all age groups if *S. aureus* suspected, additional cloxacillin or co-amoxiclav as first line and vancomycin as second line.
  - De-escalation to oral antibiotics: when the child has become afebrile with subsidence of fast breathing and increased work of breathing, switch over to oral amoxicillin and the 5–7 days of antibiotic course is completed. In the case of IV cloxacillin or co-amoxiclav for staph pneumonia, switch over to oral cloxacillin or co-amoxiclav to complete 2 weeks of treatment.

This child was started on IV ceftriaxone. She was off oxygen by day 2. Tachypnea and increased work of breathing settled on day 3 along with resolution of her fever, and she started taking oral feeds.

11. *What are the complications of pneumonia?*

The complications that may occur include:

Respiratory failure can occur requiring ICU care and ventilatory support.

Septic shock can occur in the acute stage. Supportive care with inotropes and ventilation may be required. Toxin-mediated infection such as due to *S. aureus* should be suspected and appropriate antibiotics with anti-toxin effect should be initiated.

Parapneumonic effusion/empyema can occur with any bacterial etiology but is more common with *S. aureus* or *S. pneumoniae* infection. Small effusions subside with antibiotic therapy alone. A moderate to large effusion should be suspected if the clinical improvement does not occur in 2–3 days of appropriate antibiotic therapy

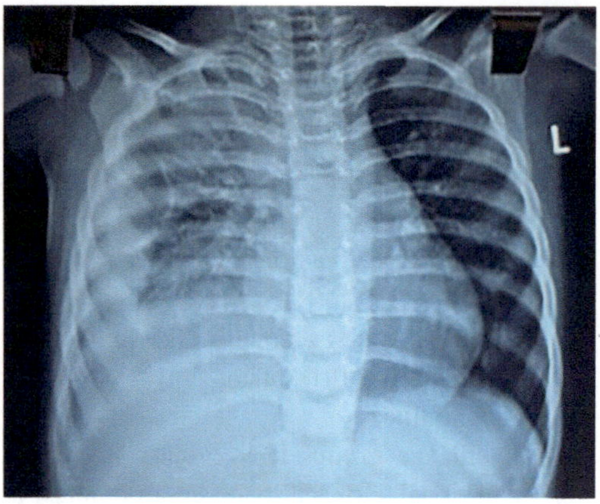

Fig. 3.2 Right-sided pneumonia with effusion (Photo courtesy Dr. Rohit Agarwal)

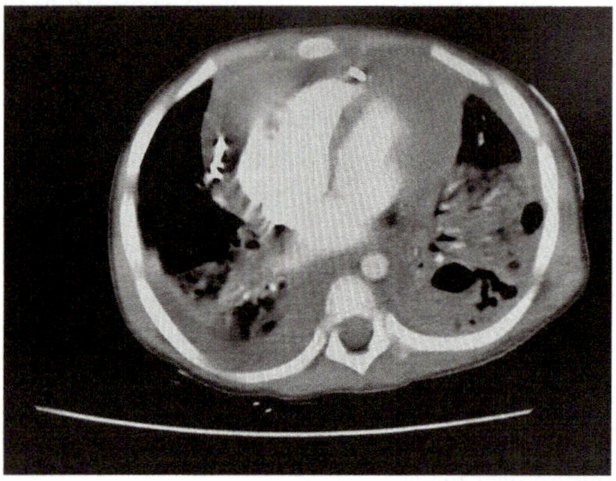

Fig. 3.3 CT showing bilateral necrotizing pneumonia (Photo courtesy Dr. Rohit Agarwal)

(Fig. 3.2). Lung USG is a useful modality to assess the extent and nature of pleural effusion as well as the development of loculations and septations in pleural space. Repeated aspiration or a chest tube placement may be required. Sometimes surgical extirpation of thick peel of pleura by video-assisted or open thoracotomy may be required.

Necrotizing pneumonia (Fig. 3.3): Necrosis of the lung tissue with cavity formation may occur. This is seen mainly with *S. pneumoniae* infection and rarely with *S. aureus* or *Klebsiella pneumoniae*. The treatment is a prolonged course of antibiotic for 4 weeks.

Lung abscess: Treatment of lung abscess requires a prolonged course of antibiotic therapy for a total of 3–4 weeks. Antibiotic therapy can be changed to the oral route once the child has improved.

3.2 Conclusion

The child was discharged on day 5 with a final diagnosis of community acquired pneumonia left upper lobe with advice to take 2 more days of oral amoxicillin. The child was reviewed after 1 week and was doing well.

Learning Points

1. In young infants, pneumonia may present as fever without a focus and irritability without cough.
2. Community acquired pneumonia (CAP) is a leading cause of under 5 mortality and morbidity and can be due to viruses or bacteria.
3. Respiratory syncytial virus (RSV) and *Streptococcus pneumoniae* are the leading causative organisms among the viruses and bacteria, respectively. With the universal Hib and PCV use, viruses are seen to be the main causative organisms in CAP.
4. Identification of the exact causative organism may not be possible on clinical and radiological features, though there may be clues.
5. A chest X-ray is recommended only for inpatients.
6. Lung ultrasound if available serves as an excellent mode to not only diagnose pneumonia but also to recognize complications such as pleural effusion.
7. Besides diagnosing pneumonia, the clinical examination aims to classify it as pneumonia and severe pneumonia. This is essential to decide management.
8. In a child with cough, *pneumonia* is diagnosed with tachypnea and/or diffi-

cult breathing and *severe pneumonia* is diagnosed when general danger signs are present.

9. Children with pneumonia are treated with oral amoxicillin, while those with severe pneumonia and children less than 3 months are treated with parenteral antibiotics.
10. Triaging a sick child with pneumonia is important to identify respiratory distress and respiratory failure so that emergency interventions can be taken to stabilize the child.

Suggested Readings

Farooqui H, Jit M, Heymann DL, Zodpey S. Burden of severe pneumonia, pneumococcal pneumonia and pneumonia deaths in Indian states: modelling based estimates. PLoS One. 2015;10(6):e0129191. https://doi.org/10.1371/journal.pone.0129191.

Ministry of Health and Family Welfare, Government of India. Introduction of pneumococcal conjugate vaccine (PCV): National Operational Guidelines. 2017. https://nhm.gov.in/New_Updates_2018/NHM_Components/Immunization/Guildelines_for_immunization/Operational_Guidelines_for_PCV_introduction.pdf. Accessed 15 Apr 2024.

Pneumonia Etiology Research for Child Health (PERCH) Study Group. Causes of severe pneumonia requiring hospital admission in children without HIV infection from Africa and Asia: the PERCH multi-country case-control study. Lancet. 2019;394:757–79.

Pneumonia in children—World Health Organization (WHO). www.who.int/news-room/fact-sheets/detail/pneumonia. Downloaded 30 March 2024.

Wahl B, Knoll MD, Shet A, et al. National, regional, and state-level pneumonia and severe pneumonia morbidity in children in India: modelled estimates for 2000 and 2015. Lancet Child Adolesc Health. 2020;4:678–87.

Dengue Fever

4

Contents

> **Key Messages**
> Dengue fever should be suspected in every febrile child from an endemic area, even when they present with gastrointestinal or respiratory symptoms. Infants with dengue fever are at high risk of severe disease and should always be hospitalized and monitored.

4.1 Case Discussion

A 7-month-old baby girl, without any relevant prior medical history, was brought to the hospital with a 2-day history of fever; the fever was abrupt in onset and continuous with a maximum temperature of 103.4F. The child also had a history of coryza and occasional cough. There was no family history of a similar illness. The child was feeding well and had a urine output as usual. Physical examination was normal.

1. *What should be done for this baby?*

This child has a fever with mild respiratory symptoms. In view of high temperature, the differential diagnosis should include bacterial and viral infections. In children who have received the primary series of three immunizations with conjugate vaccines against *Streptococcus pneumoniae* and *Haemophilus influenzae* type b, occult urinary tract infection (UTI) is the most common bacterial infection. Viral respiratory illness is suspected if there is a family history of similar illness. In view of high fever, a complete blood count and urine routine and culture should be sent, and the child should be reviewed with the report.

She was diagnosed with probable upper respiratory tract infection and prescribed paracetamol and investigated according to the plan. The child came back after 48 h with continued fever. The child was accepting and retaining breast feeds but was not playful. On examination, the vital signs and hydration were normal; the child appeared flushed (Fig. 4.1) but there were no rashes and physical examination continued to be normal.

P. Venkat Ramanan, R. Padmanabhan, *Fever in Children*,
https://doi.org/10.1007/978-981-97-9967-1_4

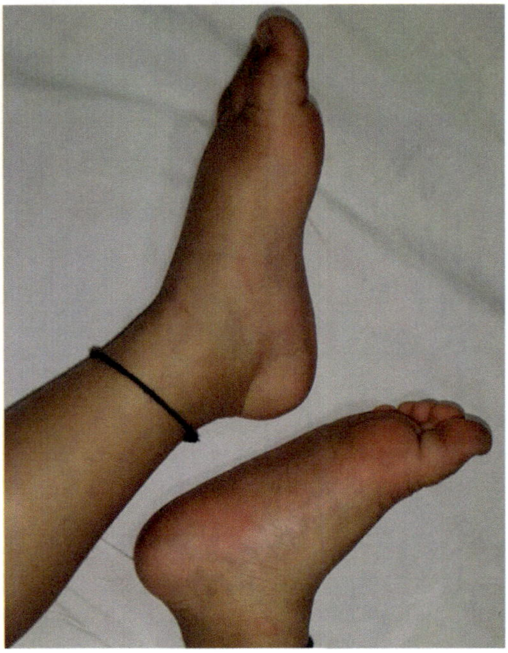

Fig. 4.1 Soles of the infant showing flushing (Photo courtesy Dr. P. Rajakumar)

The initial laboratory data revealed: hemoglobin (Hb) 11.2 g/dL, hematocrit (Hct) 33.6%, white blood cell count (WBC) 3400/mm,^{3} absolute neutrophil count (ANC) 1452/mm^3, platelets 115,000/mm^3, and C-reactive protein (CRP) 0.6 mg/dL. Urine routine was normal and culture showed no growth.

2. *What should be done now?*

As the infant is not active and fever has been persisting for 4 days, she should be hospitalized for monitoring and hydration and the investigations should be repeated. UTI has been ruled out and the normal CRP makes other bacterial infections less likely. Flushing is a feature of dengue fever. Leukopenia with thrombocytopenia should raise the suspicion of infections such as dengue, typhoid fever, and malaria in malaria-endemic areas, but such typical changes may not be seen in these infections all the time. In typhoid, neutrophilia is seen along with leukopenia. Thrombocytopenia in dengue may not be seen in the first 3–4 days.

3. *What is dengue fever and when should dengue fever be suspected?*

Dengue fever, endemic in our country, is an infection caused by the dengue virus which has four serotypes, namely DENV-1, DENV-2, DENV-3, and DENV-4. The virus is transmitted through the bites of infected *Aedes aegypti* mosquitoes. The spectrum of clinical manifestations varies, and the presentation ranges from undifferentiated fever, dengue fever (DF), dengue fever with warning signs and severe dengue, to Expanded Dengue Syndrome.

Dengue fever in infants is challenging to recognize because of its presentation with gastrointestinal and upper respiratory symptoms that are similar to other viral illness. Hence, one must have a high index of suspicion. It is important to suspect dengue fever in every febrile child from the endemic areas, particularly if thrombocytopenia, leukopenia, flushing, and/or rashes are present.

Typically, dengue fever has three phases: the febrile phase, lasting for 3–7 days, during which there is fever which may be bi-phasic and associated with headache, body pain, flushing, and a maculopapular rash . The critical phase is between days 4 and 7, usually when the fever resolves. The "warning signs" in dengue fever include abdominal pain or tenderness, persistent vomiting, clinical fluid accumulation (Figs. 4.2 and 4.3), mucosal bleed, lethargy, restlessness, and liver enlargement. The capillary leak and abnormal hemostasis that occur during this phase may lead to shock and internal bleeding (severe dengue). The convalescent phase (recovery phase) follows the critical phase. The fluid that has leaked out of the capillaries returns to the circulation and the signs and symptoms resolve.

4. *What are the tests to be done in suspected dengue fever?*

During the early stages of the disease (first 4–5 days of fever), there is viremia, and dengue NS1 antigen can be detected in the blood to diagnose the infection. After day 5 of fever, serology is the method of choice for diagnosis. IgM antibodies are the first to appear. These antibodies are detect-

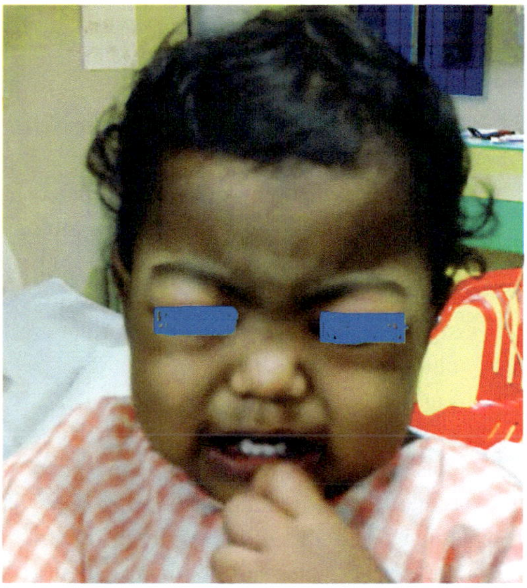

Fig. 4.2 Periorbital fluffiness due to capillary leak (Photo courtesy Dr. P. Rajakumar)

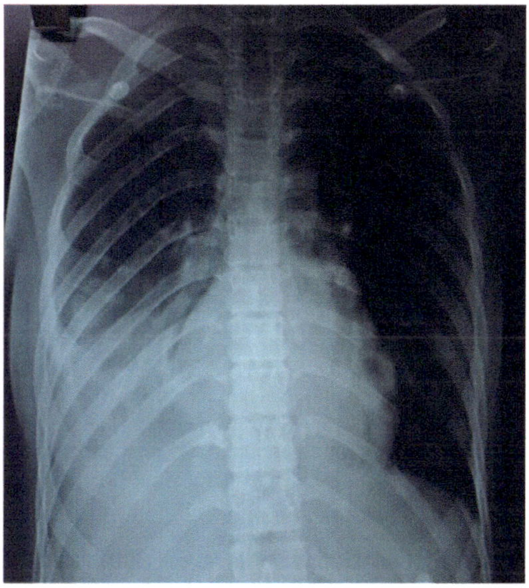

Fig. 4.3 Chest X-ray showing right pleural effusion due to capillary leak (Photo courtesy Dr. P. Rajakumar)

able in 50% of patients by days 3–5 after fever onset, in 80% by day 5, and in 99% by day 10. IgM levels peak about 2 weeks after fever onset and then decline, becoming undetectable after 2–3 months. Anti-dengue serum IgG antibodies are generally detectable at low titers by the end of the first week, increasing slowly thereafter, and remain detectable for several months, probably even for life. During a secondary dengue infection, the dominant immunoglobulin isotype is IgG even in the acute phase, and IgM levels are significantly lower. To distinguish between primary and secondary dengue infections, the IgM/IgG antibody ratios are now more commonly used.

In suspected dengue fever, a baseline hematocrit is important. An increase in the hematocrit by 20% from the baseline is an indicator of hemoconcentration due to plasma leak. In addition, a coagulation profile and liver function test would also help in assessing the severity of the illness, especially if there are warning signs. Low platelet count is a universal finding after the fourth day of fever. Although minor bleeding may occur, severe bleeding is uncommon unless the course is complicated with severe shock and multiorgan failure. Hemoconcentration is less easily identified in our country, probably because of the underlying nutritional anemia prevalent among the children.

The infant was hospitalized and blood investigations were sent. Laboratory results on day 4 of fever showed the following: hemoglobin 12.2 g/dL, hematocrit 36.6%, leukocytes 2900/mm^3 and platelets 86,000/ mm^3, PTT 63 s (control 24 s), and PT 18.6 s (control 15.2 s). Dengue NS1Ag and serology for IgM antibodies against dengue were positive.

5. *What should be done now?*

The management of dengue fever is primarily supportive, maintaining hydration and early detection of complications.

Vital signs such as pulse rate, respiratory rate, capillary refill time (CRT), (The term capillary refill time [CRT] is used for uniformity) and blood pressure should be checked at least every 4 h in non-shock patients and 1–2 h in shock patients. Serial checking of hematocrit every 6 h is important to detect plasma leak. Urine output should be recorded at least every 8–12 h in uncomplicated cases and on an hourly basis in patients with shock or fluid overload. The urine output should be about 0.5 mL/kg/h.

Oral feeding was encouraged and as there was infrequent wetting of the diapers, the infant was catheterized to monitor her urine output.

The fever persisted and at 24 h of hospitalization she became drowsy and was refusing oral feeding. Her urine output was 0.4 mL/kg/h and capillary refill time (CFT) was 3 s. The hemoglobin was 13.6 g/dL, hematocrit 40.8% (21.4% rise compared to the baseline hematocrit of 33.6), and platelet count 32,000/mm^3. Intravenous crystalloids were administered according to the WHO protocol and her urine output and CFT improved. However, 12 h later, she was found to have cold peripheries and her CFT was again prolonged. She also developed petechiae and ecchymosis. She was shifted to the intensive care unit, resuscitated with crystalloids, and closely monitored.

6. *Why did this child deteriorate in spite of hospitalization and initiation of treatment?*

In children, especially during the critical phase of illness, there is minute-to-minute variation in the clinical illness state. Some children may go in and out of shock a few times during the critical phase. Continuous monitoring helps in recognizing shock early (compensated shock) before the blood pressure drops and hypoperfusion develops. It is important to examine the infant repeatedly for cold peripheries and prolonged CRT to identify shock early. Hypotension is a late sign. Narrowing of pulse pressure to <20 mmHg is an early feature of shock in dengue. Infants 4–9 months of age are particularly vulnerable to complications. Because of antibody-dependent enhancement, infants born to mothers with past dengue infection are at risk of more severe disease when infected with a different DENV strain. Manifestations such as convulsions and hepatic dysfunction are also more common among infants than in older children, and the fatality rate is four times higher in infants.

4.2 Conclusion

The patient improved hemodynamically with fluid management in the intensive care. She was then shifted to the ward after 24 h, observed, and discharged after a day.

Learning Points

1. Dengue fever is one of the most common causes of "undifferentiated tropical fevers" in children in India.
2. Dengue fever in children is associated with higher morbidity and mortality especially in infants.
3. Parental education about the warning signs and when to return is important in outpatient management.
4. Early diagnosis, adherence to the recommended clinical management protocols, and close monitoring can help reduce the case fatality ratio.
5. Infants with dengue fever are at risk of more severe diseases and hence should be hospitalized during the critical phase and closely monitored.
6. Clinical examination of cold peripheries and prolonged CRT and monitoring the urine output are the best methods to identify shock early. Hypotension is a late sign.

Suggested Readings

Dash N, Aby R, Kumar M, Abraham AM, Rose W. Infant dengue a 10-year experience from a tertiary Center in South India. Am J Trop Med Hyg. 2021;105(2):435–9. https://doi.org/10.4269/ajtmh.21-0159. PMID: 34237019; PMCID: PMC8437169.

Directorate General of Health Services, Ministry of Health and Family Welfare, Government of India. 2020. National Guideline for Dengue Case Management during COVID-19 Pandemic. [Online]. https://nvbdcp.gov.in/Doc/National%20Guideline%20for%20Dengue%20case%20management%20during%20COVID-19%20pandemic.pdf. Accessed Dec 2023.

World health Organization. Comprehensive guideline for prevention and control of dengue and dengue Haemorrhagic fever. New Delhi: World Health Organization, Regional Office for South-East Asia; 2011.

Scrub Typhus

5

Contents

> **Key Messages**
> Scrub typhus is one of the re-emerging tropical infections, and it should be considered in the differential diagnosis of any child with fever for more than 5 days. The presence of an eschar is diagnostic, hence the need for a diligent physical examination. Empirical doxycycline therapy may be life-saving in appropriate clinical settings.

5.1 Case Discussion

An 8-year-old boy, previously well, was brought with a history of fever for 5 days, headache, myalgia, and decreased appetite. His body temperature was always >100 °F with the maximum temperature touching 104 °F. There were no respiratory or gastrointestinal symptoms. He was seen by a private practitioner on day 2 of illness and was prescribed paracetamol. As the fever persisted, he approached another doctor on day 4 of fever and was advised to take cefixime and to continue paracetamol. His symptoms persisted and on day 4 of illness, and he developed mild facial puffiness and a non-itchy skin rash. He was passing clear urine, in adequate amounts. There was occasional abdominal pain and the stools were normal. He resided in a semiurban area, and there is no recent travel history. He was studying in third standard, and there was no significant illness in the past. His parents and one elder brother were well.

On examination, the boy was febrile and well oriented, but looked ill. He had facial puffiness and pedal edema. There were bilateral cervical lymph nodes of 1.5–2 cm, bilateral axillary nodes of 1–1.5 cm, and a few inguinal lymph nodes of 1 cm. All the nodes were nontender. There was no pallor or icterus. His body temperature was 103 °F, pulse rate 120/min, respiratory rate 28/min, and blood pressure 100/70 mmHg. He had conjunctival injection, and the oral cavity and throat were normal. A maculopapular rash was present over the trunk and extremities with sparing of palms and soles. A thorough head to foot examination did not reveal any other skin lesion.

P. Venkat Ramanan, R. Padmanabhan, *Fever in Children*,
https://doi.org/10.1007/978-981-97-9967-1_5

On systemic examination, the liver was palpable 6 cm below right costal margin, and it was smooth and not tender. The spleen tip was palpable. On auscultation, cardiovascular system and respiratory system were normal.

1. *What are the possibilities in a child with fever for 5 days, rash, generalized lymphadenopathy, and hepatosplenomegaly (HSM)?*

There are many infectious and noninfectious conditions that can have such a presentation. The infectious causes include viruses (dengue, Epstein–Barr virus (EBV), chikungunya), bacteria (leptospirosis, enteric fever, scarlet fever, meningococcemia), mycoplasma, rickettsiae (scrub typhus, spotted fever group), and toxic shock syndrome. The noninfectious causes include allergies (drug hypersensitivity) and Kawasaki disease (KD). Beyond 10–14 days of fever, connective tissue disorders, tuberculosis and malignancies should also be considered.

Dengue fever, enteric fever, scrub typhus (a type of rickettsial infection), and EBV infection are the main differentials in this child. Puffiness of face with pedal edema is characteristic of conditions associated with vasculitis such as dengue fever and rickettsial infection. Dengue is a very common infection and occurs round the year. The fever in dengue does not last for more than 7 days unless a complication such as hemophagocytic lymphohistiocytosis (HLH) sets in. Enteric fever must always be considered in an endemic country like India in any fever lasting beyond 5 days. The typical rose spots described in 15–30% of cases of enteric fever in Western textbooks are hardly ever seen in Indian children, probably due to the darker skin complexion and the evanescent nature of rash.

Chikungunya is usually associated with arthritis/arthralgia. The presence of exudative tonsillitis or icterus may point toward EBV infection. In toxic shock syndrome, usually secondary to streptococcal or staphylococcal infection of skin and soft tissues, the child will be quite ill with sudden onset of high-grade fever and hypotension. The cervical lymphadenopathy in KD is characteristically unilateral. The absence of mucosal changes and the age of >5 years make KD less likely in this child.

Scrub typhus was considered more likely in this child in view of persistent fever with edema, generalized rash, lymphadenopathy, and hepatosplenomegaly .

The child was hospitalized and investigated. His blood reports revealed a hemoglobin of 11.6 g/dL (Normal 11.5–14.5 g/dL); total leukocyte count (TLC) 7040/cmm (4000–12,000/cmm), differential leucocyte count (DLC) showed neutrophils 77.8% (54–62%), lymphocytes 20% (25–33%), eosinophils 0 (1–3%), monocytes 1.6% (3–7%), and basophils 0.6% (0–0.75%); and platelet count was 150,000/cmm (150,000–400,000/cmm). Peripheral smear for malarial parasite was negative. Liver function tests revealed a total serum protein of 6.2 g/dL (6.4–8.1 g/dL), albumin of 2.8 g/dL (3.5–5.6 g/dL) and globulin of 3.4 g/dL, serum aspartate aminotransferase (AST) or glutamic oxaloacetic transaminase (SGOT) level of 55 units/L (normal: 15–50 units/L), and serum alanine aminotransferase (ALT) or glutamic-pyruvic transaminase (SGPT) level of 65 units/L (normal: 5–45 units/L). Serum bilirubin was 0.8 mg/dL. C-reactive protein was 8 mg/dL (normal <0.6 mg/dL). Serum electrolyte estimation revealed sodium of 130mMol/L, potassium of 4.8mMol/L, and chloride of 104mMol/L. Blood urea nitrogen (BUN) was 12 mg/dL (5–18 mg/dL), and serum creatinine was 0.4 mg/dL (0.22–0.59 mg/dL). Blood was sent for culture and sensitivity and serology for dengue, and IgM ELISA for scrub typhus and leptospirosis.

2. *Should you start this child on any empirical treatment?*

Specific treatment is available only for bacterial infections. The common bacterial infections to be suspected in this child are enteric fever, scrub typhus, and leptospirosis. These bacterial infections also may lead to complications in the second week of infection if not treated. Hence, empirical treatment with a third-generation cephalosporin and doxycycline targeting these infections is recommended after sending the appropriate blood samples for investigation. Among the noninfective causes, vasculitis such as Kawasaki disease needs to be suspected, as the delay in initiating treatment in KD can lead to serious coronary artery disease.

This child was started on IV ceftriaxone and oral doxycycline as empirical therapy for enteric fever and scrub typhus, respectively. Supportive care such as adequate hydration and paracetamol for fever was also instituted. On the second day of hospitalization, IgM ELISA for scrub typhus was reported as positive. IgM ELISA for leptospirosis and dengue serology was negative. Later, blood culture report also turned out to be negative.

3. *What is scrub typhus and how frequently is it seen as a cause of fever in children?*

Scrub typhus is one of the re-emerging tropical infections and is caused by *Orientia tsutsugamushi*, a Gram-negative intracellular coccobacillus. It belongs to the rickettsial group. Rickettsial infections are classified into four groups: (1) spotted fever, (2) typhus, (3) scrub typhus, and (4) miscellaneous. Nearly 90% of the rickettsial infections in India are due to scrub typhus, and it is seen throughout the country in all age groups both in rural and urban areas. The remaining 10% of cases are the spotted fever group of Indian tick typhus seen in some parts of the country such as Karnataka, Maharashtra, and Tamil Nadu. Both respond to the same group of antibiotics. Scrub typhus is a mite-borne zoonotic infection. The larval forms of the trombiculid mites (known as chiggers) of the genus *Leptotrombidium* are the vectors as well as the reservoirs. The incubation period is 7–10 days following the bite of the larval mite.

4. *What are the clinical features of scrub typhus?*

Scrub typhus is an acute febrile infection seen in all age groups. Abrupt onset of high fever, anorexia, headache, myalgia, and arthralgia are characteristic. Cough, ocular pain, and conjunctival injection may be seen. Some children may have significant gastrointestinal symptoms such as vomiting, diarrhea, and abdominal pain. Mostly, the initial clinical presentation is that of any undifferentiated fever such as dengue, enteric fever, or malaria. In some children, maculopapular rash develops 48–72 h after the fever onset and is seen over the trunk, extremities, and face, sparing the palms and soles. The rash is more common in spotted fever (Indian tick typhus), and the palms and soles are also usually involved. In scrub typhus, a characteristic skin lesion known as "eschar" is seen.

Eschar is a painless well-circumscribed papule with central necrosis with or without a black crust characteristic of scrub typhus (Fig. 5.1) and is reported in 7–97% of cases. Its specificity for diagnosis of scrub typhus is nearly 100%. It occurs at the site of chigger bite and is usually single, measuring 0.5 cm to 1 cm and is present most commonly in skin folds. A thorough physical examination including the axilla, gluteal cleft, behind the ears, and the groin is essential, otherwise it may be missed. Asking the mother or the child himself if any new skin ulcer has appeared may also be helpful.

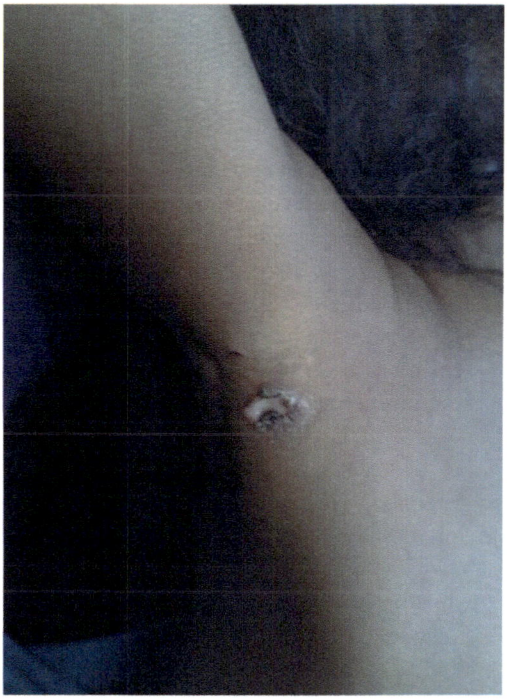

Fig. 5.1 Eschar of scrub typhus in the right axilla

Lymphadenopathy: Localized lymphadenopathy in the draining area of eschar and generalized lymphadenopathy are commonly seen.

Edema: Periorbital puffiness and pedal edema may be seen 2–4 days after the onset of fever due to the generalized vascular leak as the organism mainly affects the vascular endothelium.

The triad of fever, rash, and edema should raise the suspicion of scrub typhus and the presence of eschar confirms it.

Systemic features: Along with fever and the aforementioned manifestations, respiratory, gastrointestinal, and neurologic involvement can occur. Respiratory involvement can start with cough and progressively worsen to respiratory distress. Neurologic presentation may be in the form of meningitis or acute encephalitis. Scrub typhus has been found to be a common cause of acute encephalitic syndrome in children. Going into second week, untreated scrub typhus can result in severe organ involvement and death.

5. *What are the investigations that help in the diagnosis of scrub typhus?*

The diagnosis mainly rests on serological tests, which become positive after day 5–7 of illness. The tests employed for scrub typhus are as follows:

1. **IgM ELISA:** It is a serologic test commonly performed in many laboratories in our country and has high sensitivity and specificity.
2. **Weil Felix test**: Agglutination titer of 1:80–1:320 is considered positive. It is economic and technically easy to do. It has a poor sensitivity though the specificity is good.
3. **Immunofluorescent assay (IFA)**: This test is considered the "gold" standard, but it is costlier and technically demanding, and is not generally available.
4. **Polymerase chain reaction (PCR)**: The sensitivity of PCR ranges from 22.5% to 82%, while the specificity is near 100% especially in the first week of illness when the serology is negative. It can be done in blood as well as in the eschar scrapings. It is available only in some centers.
5. **Culture of the organism**: This is also available only in specialized laboratories.

6. *What are the other laboratory tests that may suggest scrub typhus?*

Though other laboratory parameters are not definitive, they may offer some clues to suspect scrub typhus (Box 5.1). Some of the findings may overlap with other viral infections, dengue fever, malaria, and enteric fever.

Box 5.1 Other Nonspecific Lab Findings in Scrub Typhus

- TLC: Normal or low, later may increase.
- Platelets decreased (true reduction or pseudo thrombocytopenia due to platelet aggregates which can be made out in peripheral smear).
- Increased ESR/CRP.
- Decreased serum albumin.
- Decreased serum sodium.
- Raised liver enzymes such as ALT, AST.

This child showed normal WBC counts and platelets, increased CRP, decreased serum albumin, elevated liver enzyme levels, and decreased serum sodium.

7. *What is the treatment for scrub typhus?*

Though the diagnosis is difficult in the initial phase of infection, early treatment based on the epidemiology and suggestive clinical and laboratory features helps in prompt recovery. Identifying an eschar is helpful in making an early specific diagnosis. Each day of delay in treatment as the child goes into the second week of fever is fraught with the danger of multiple complications. Response to appropriate antibiotics is dramatic with the fever subsiding in 24–48 h of initiating antibiotic therapy. This therapeutic response can prove to be a diagnostic test, and one can think of an alternative diagnosis if fever does not subside. The commonly used drugs for scrub typhus are doxycycline, azithromycin, chloramphenicol, and rifampicin. Doxycycline is the drug of choice. It can be used in all age groups and in pregnancy as well.

Doxycycline: 2.2 mg/kg/dose orally (PO) or intravenously (IV) twice daily for children <45 kg and 100 mg PO or IV twice daily for those weighing ≥45 kg. The treatment is given for 7 days or up to 3 days after defervescence of fever.

Azithromycin: May be required if there is allergy to doxycycline. It can be given orally or IV. Oral dose is 10 mg/kg/day for 5 days.

Chloramphenicol: Not used nowadays in view of availability of effective alternate drugs with less toxicity.

Rifampicin: May be useful in the rare event of doxycycline resistance. It is not to be used routinely for the treatment of scrub typhus in India as it is an important first-line drug for tuberculosis.

IV preparations of doxycycline or azithromycin are used in complicated cases.

8. *What are the complications of scrub typhus?*

Severe complications may develop in untreated scrub typhus, usually in the second week of illness. CNS complications (ranging from aseptic meningitis to acute meningoencephalitis), acute respiratory distress syndrome (ARDS), myocarditis, acute renal failure, disseminated intravascular coagulation (DIC), shock and multi-organ dysfunction syndrome (MODS) may develop. Mortality up to 35% can occur when untreated or treatment is delayed.

5.2 Conclusion

A final diagnosis of scrub typhus was made. The child responded well to oral doxycycline and fever subsided in 48 h. He was discharged on the fourth day off admission, and doxycycline was given for a total duration of 5 days. He was followed up after 2 weeks and was normal.

Learning Points

1. Scrub typhus is a re-emerging tropical infection caused by a rickettsial organism transmitted by the bite of the larval form of mite.
2. It is seen in all ages and all over the country.
3. It should be considered in the differential diagnosis of any fever persisting beyond 5–7 days especially when accompanied with a maculopapular rash, edema, and lymphadenopathy.
4. Some children may have respiratory, gastrointestinal, or neurological manifestations.
5. The presence of an eschar clinches the diagnosis of scrub typhus, hence the importance of a diligent search for an eschar as it may be hidden in the crevices and folds of the body.
6. IgM ELISA is the diagnostic test of choice done after 5 days of fever.
7. PCR test of blood or eschar scrapings though diagnostic in the first week of illness is not easily available.
8. Empiric treatment should be initiated in suspected cases without waiting for test results as the delay may be associated with severe complications.
9. Doxycycline is the drug of choice and can be used at all ages.
10. Complications such as acute meningoencephalitis, ARDS, myocarditis, acute renal failure, DIC, shock, and multi-organ dysfunction syndrome can occur in the second week of illness.

Suggested Readings

Lo SF. Reference intervals for laboratory tests and procedures. In: Kliegman RM, Stanton BF, St Geme JW, Schor NF, editors. Nelson textbook 1st South Asia edition. New Delhi: Reed Elsevier India Pvt Ltd; 2016. p. 3464–72.

Rapsang AG, Bhattcharyya P. Scrub typhus. Indian J Anaesth. 2013;57:127–34.

Rathi N, Kulkarni A, Yewale V. For Indian Academy of Pediatrics IAP Guidelines on Rickettsial Diseases in Children. Ind Pediatr. 2017;5:223–9.

Enteric Fever

6

Contents

> **Key Messages**
> Enteric fever should be considered in the differential diagnosis of children with fever and diarrhea if the fever persists for over 5 days. In our country, enteric fever is not uncommon in young children including infants.

6.1 Case Discussion

A 14-month-old boy was brought by his parents with a history of fever with vomiting for 3 days and watery diarrhea for 2 days. The maximum body temperature was 101.4 F. There was no blood or mucus in the stool. He was previously healthy with no significant past medical history. He had received all the IAP recommended vaccines till date including the typhoid conjugate vaccine. On examination, his hydration was normal and no other focus of infection was found.

1. *What would be the clinical diagnosis and management of this child?*

The clinical diagnosis would be acute watery diarrhea (AWD) with no dehydration. Other possibilities that need to be considered are urinary tract infection and dengue fever as the occurrence of diarrhea does not exclude these common conditions. On the third day of fever when there is a focus of infection (diarrhea), whether to undertake laboratory investigations in all children is a difficult decision.

Acute watery diarrhoea (AWD) is usually caused by viruses like rotavirus and less commonly by bacteria and parasites. It is self-limiting, no investigations are indicated, and the management focuses on maintaining hydration. The WHO recommends zinc supplementation for children under 5 years of age: at a dose of 20 mg/day for children older than 6 months or 10 mg/day in those younger than 6 months for 14 days. Ondansetron can help in controlling vomiting. When there is no blood or mucus in the stool, there is no role of antibiotics.

P. Venkat Ramanan, R. Padmanabhan, *Fever in Children*,
https://doi.org/10.1007/978-981-97-9967-1_6

As the child was taking and retaining feeds and the general condition appeared normal, a diagnosis of AWD was made, and it was decided to closely follow-up the child. Oral rehydration solution, zinc, and paracetamol were started. The warning signs of dehydration and danger signs of dengue were explained, and the parents were advised to return if the expected improvement did not occur in 2 days or any time if danger sign(s) developed to test for other infections such as urinary tract infection (UTI), dengue, and typhoid fever.

2. *This child had received three doses of rotavirus vaccine. Could he still get the infection?*

The available studies in India and other Asian neighboring countries indicate that the vaccine offers about 50% protection from severe rotavirus illness needing hospitalization. So it is still possible to get the infection after taking three doses of rotavirus vaccine.

The child was brought to the clinic after 3 days (sixth day of fever onset) with complaints of persisting high-grade fever despite the medication provided. The loose stools had subsided but vomiting off and on persisted. On examination, he was found to be lethargic and irritable, and showed signs of some dehydration. The pulse rate was 120 beats/min, and the axillary temperature was 104.2 °F. There were no new findings on examination or evidence of hepatosplenomegaly.

3. *What is the cause of persistent fever despite loose stools resolving and how should we proceed?*

In rotaviral diarrhea, typically, the early symptoms are fever and vomiting, followed by 3–7 days of watery diarrhea. With fever persisting after resolution of diarrhea, the possibility of other infections such as UTI, dengue, enteric fever, scrub typhus, influenza, chikungunya, COVID-19, and other viral infections should be considered. Of these, UTI, enteric fever, and scrub typhus require specific antimicrobial therapy.

This child should be hospitalized, investigated for the conditions listed above, and started on parenteral antibiotics after sending cultures.

The child was managed as described above and started on intravenous injection of ceftriaxone 100 mg/kg/day in two divided doses. Laboratory investigations showed a hemoglobin of 11.9 g/dL (normal 11–14.5 g/dL), total leucocyte count (TLC) of 3160 cells/mm^3 (normal 3200–9800 cells/mm^3) with a differential count of 49% neutrophils (normal 54–62%); 0.1% eosinophils (normal 1–3%), 4.8% monocytes (normal 3–7%), 0.3% basophils (normal <1%), 43% lymphocytes (normal: 25–33%), and a platelet count of 145,000/mm^3 (normal: 130000–400,000 cells/mm^3). The serum glutamic oxaloacetic transaminase (SGOT) level was 88 units/L (normal: 0–35 units/L), serum glutamic-pyruvic transaminase (SGPT) level was 95 units/L (normal value: 0–35 units/L), erythrocyte sedimentation rate (ESR) was 9 mm/h (normal value: 0–20 mm/h), and C-reactive protein was 2.26 mg/dL (normal <0.6 mg/dL).

On day 3 of hospitalization, the blood culture was reported to be growing *Salmonella enterica* serovar Paratyphi A (*S.* Paratyphi A).

4. *What is enteric fever?*

Infection with gram-negative bacteria *Salmonella typhi* (*S. typhi*) and Paratyphi A and B is collectively known as enteric fever. *S. typhi* is the most common cause of enteric fever globally, and paratyphoid is seen mostly in South Asia and China with *S.* Paratyphi A being the dominant cause of paratyphoid fever in South Asia. Both typhoid and paratyphoid infections are caused by ingestion of food or water contaminated by infected human feces and is mostly seen in children without access to clean drinking water and proper sanitation.

5. *When should enteric fever be suspected as the cause of fever?*

Symptoms start 7–14 days after exposure (range 3–60 days). Paratyphoid fever has a shorter incubation period (4–5 days), but symptoms are indistinguishable from those of typhoid fever.

A fever of gradual onset that persists for over 5 days, particularly with gastrointestinal symptoms like diarrhea, vomiting, and abdominal pain, should raise the suspicion of enteric fever in children from endemic regions or with a history of travel to endemic regions. Diarrhea is more commonly seen in children, while constipation is common in adults with enteric fever. The fever typically rises to a plateau of 39–40 °C (102–104 °F) toward the end of the first week. Patients may also have headache, cough, and malaise. Children under 5 years of age frequently present with only fever, and the diagnosis may be missed unless they have complications.

The physical findings are often nonspecific: a coated tongue, abdominal distension, and a diffuse or localized tenderness may be noted. A tender hepatomegaly is seen in up to 85% and splenomegaly in 90% of children under 5 years by the end of 1 week. Scattered wheezes or crepitations in the chest might suggest bronchitis. A bradycardia relative to the height of the fever may be noted. Rose spots, blanching erythematous maculopapular lesions on the trunk, were considered characteristic of typhoid fever but are now rarely reported.

Clinical diagnosis of enteric fever is difficult as symptoms overlap with other causes of fever.

6. *What are the investigations that help in making a diagnosis?*

The clinician should always send the blood for culture before starting empiric antibiotic therapy for enteric fever. Blood culture is the gold standard for diagnosis by isolating the organism and testing antimicrobial sensitivity. However, its sensitivity is only around 61%. Antibiotic pretreatment, low sample volume, and low circulating bacterial load in the blood lower the sensitivity and a negative blood culture does not exclude enteric fever. Bone marrow culture gives a higher yield, but it is rarely performed. Feces and urine may be cultured later in the course of illness, but a positive result may indicate chronic carriage rather than an acute infection.

Serological tests, including the Widal test, and the newer commercially available, point-of-care rapid diagnostic tests (RDT) are not useful in diagnosis. The Widal test measures antibodies against O and H antigens of *S. typhi* and *S.* Paratyphi A. It is cheap and simple but lacks sensitivity and specificity and is not recommended. The Typhidot test that detects IgM and IgG antibodies against the outer membrane proteins (OMP) of *S. typhi* has an average sensitivity of 66% (59–73%) with a specificity of 81% (58–93%) across a number of versions.

The other blood tests may give a clue. *Salmonella* is an intracellular organism, and it induces apoptosis in the macrophages that it infects and leukopenia is common in older children. Eosinopenia, seen in up to 70% of children with enteric fever, is an important indicator of disease severity. In children under 5, leukocytosis or a normal leukocyte count is more common. Leukocytosis in older children suggests complication of enteric fever such as intestinal perforation or another diagnosis such as a pyogenic infection or leptospirosis. A mild normochromic or hypochromic anemia, mild thrombocytopenia, and mild elevation of liver transaminases with a normal bilirubin level are also common. The C-reactive protein (CRP) is usually elevated in enteric fever.

7. *How is it treated?*

Ideally, definitive antimicrobial therapy for enteric fever should be based on the results of susceptibility testing. However, antimicrobials will have to be used empirically till the blood culture report is released and when the diagnosis is presumptive without isolation of the organism in the blood culture.

Patients can usually be managed at home if they have no complications and can tolerate oral therapy. Choice of empiric therapy depends on the antibiotic-susceptibility pattern in the geographical area where infection is acquired. For infections acquired in South Asia where there is a high prevalence of resistance to fluoroquinolones, oral azithromycin is used as it achieves excellent intracellular concentrations and has established efficacy even against XDR isolates as reported in Pakistan. Cefixime is an alternative, but a longer duration of therapy (10–14 days) is warranted because of the risk of relapse with shorter durations. If multidrug resistance is not prevalent, trimethoprim–sulfamethoxazole, amoxicillin, and chloramphenicol (if available) are potential options. Azithromycin-resistant *S. typhi* has been reported from some parts of South Asia, particularly Bangladesh.

Hospitalization is necessary if the patient is vomiting and unable to take oral medication, is clinically unstable, has developed complications, or if the diagnosis is uncertain. In such individuals, initial therapy with a parenteral agent like ceftriaxone or cefotaxime is appropriate. Concurrent treatment with doxycycline (or azithromycin in children) is advised to cover for scrub typhus and leptospirosis where these infections are endemic. Aztreonam can be used for individuals who cannot take cephalosporins because of allergy. In situations where the risk of decreased susceptibility to fluoroquinolones is low (infection acquired outside South Asia or Iraq), fluoroquinolones are an appropriate alternative. If there is suspicion for ceftriaxone resistance (history of travel to Pakistan or Iraq), carbapenem can be used till the susceptibility is known. Once the susceptibility pattern is known, de-escalation from a broad spectrum to a narrow spectrum drug is needed.

Supportive care includes ensuring adequate hydration and antipyretics for fever. High-dose corticosteroids may be considered in patients with severe disease or complications.

The general condition of the child improved over the next few days but the fever continued unabated even after 5 days of intravenous ceftriaxone.

8. *When should fever defervescence be expected after initiation of treatment with appropriate antibiotics and what is the duration of treatment?*

After initiation of treatment with cephalosporins, it generally takes 5–10 days for fever defervescence, but patients often feel better sooner as fever intervals and intensity improve. With azithromycin and ciprofloxacin, defervescence occurs in 2–7 days and 1–5 days, respectively.

If there is persistent high fever and symptoms after 7–10 days of treatment, re-evaluation is needed. Investigations including blood culture should be repeated to detect antimicrobial resistance, complications following enteric fever or another diagnosis. Azithromycin is given for 7 days. For cephalosporins, the antibiotic treatment duration of 14 days or 5 days after fever resolution, whichever is longer, is traditionally followed. Patients commenced on parenteral antimicrobials can be switched to oral medications once they are clinically stable.

9. *What are the complications?*

Complications usually manifest in the second or third week of illness. Delayed initiation of treatment, the virulence of the bacterial strain, and host factors contribute to disease severity and complications. Encephalopathy, gastrointestinal bleeding, intestinal perforation, nephritis, and hepatitis can occur. Between 5% and 10% of patients experience a relapse with a second episode of fever two to 3 weeks after initial recovery. Furthermore, 2–5% of patients, even after recovery, become asymptomatic carriers and continue to shed the bacteria.

10. *What is chronic carriage in enteric fever?*

Around 10% of adults who have had enteric fever intermittently shed bacteria in feces for several weeks after infection. If shedding continues beyond 1 year, it is called chronic carriage. Asymptomatic chronic carrier state is uncommon in children. The focus of infection in chronic carriage is thought to be the gall bladder, and carriage is more common in individuals with gall bladder disease and in women over 40 years old. Kidney stones and schistosomiasis increase the risk of persistent urinary carriage.

From the public health point of view, for food handlers and staff working in health-care or daycare facilities, three negative fecal culture samples at a minimum of 48 h apart after an acute episode of enteric fever are recommended to exclude carriage. For eradication, prolonged treatment with high dose antibiotics and, rarely, cholecystectomy may be needed. For patients with a fluoroquinolone-susceptible isolate, treatment with ciprofloxacin or levofloxacin for 4 weeks is reasonable. For patients with a fluoroquinolone-nonsusceptible isolate, treatment should be guided by susceptibility data (amoxicillin for 6 weeks or trimethoprim-sulfamethoxazole for 3 months).

11. *How can enteric fever be prevented?*

In endemic regions, improving access to clean drinking water, sanitation, high food hygiene standards, and safe sewage disposal can reduce the burden of the disease. For travelers, avoiding contaminated water, salads, ice, cold foods, and pre-travel vaccination is recommended. The World Health Organization has approved three typhoid vaccines (live oral Ty21a vaccine, parenteral Vi polysaccharide, and conjugated Vi polysaccharide vaccines), but none of them is part of the routine immunization program. There are no vaccines currently available for paratyphoid fever.

In 2018, the WHO recommended the Vi conjugate vaccine (TCV) for use in children above 6 months of age. The vaccine effectiveness is approximately 80%. Hence, there is a possibility of getting typhoid fever despite vaccination.

This child was vaccinated against typhoid, but the vaccine does not protect against *S.* Paratyphi infection.

6.2 Conclusion

Fever subsided after 9 days of antibiotic treatment. He was discharged on oral cefixime and had fully recovered on follow-up.

Learning Points

1. In endemic areas and in returning travelers, enteric fever should be considered in the differential diagnosis of fever for over 5 days, particularly if there are abdominal symptoms.
2. Blood culture is the gold standard for diagnosing enteric fever and serological tests, including the Widal test, are not recommended.
3. Antibiotic pretreatment, low sample volume, and low circulating bacterial load in the blood lower the sensitivity and a negative blood culture does not exclude enteric fever.
4. In endemic areas, for empiric treatment of fever for over 5 days, one should consider adding doxycycline (or azithromycin) for scrub typhus if third generation cephalosporin is started for suspected enteric fever.
5. The typhoid Vi conjugate vaccine is now recommended by the WHO in endemic areas for use in children above 6 months of age.
6. Even after typhoid vaccination, *S.* Paratyphi infection can cause enteric fever.
7. Antimicrobial resistance is common, so the national guidelines should be referred to for choice of antibiotic.
8. After initiation of appropriate antibiotics, fever defervescence may take 5–10 days.
9. Complications usually manifest in the second or third week of illness.

Suggested Readings

Britto C, Pollard AJ, Voysey M, Blohmke CJ. An appraisal of the clinical features of pediatric enteric fever: systematic review and meta-analysis of the age-stratified disease occurrence. Clin Infect Dis. 2017;64(11):1604–11. https://doi.org/10.1093/cid/cix229. PMID: 28369224; PMCID: PMC5434381.

Basnyat B, Qamar FN, Rupali P, Ahmed T, Parry CM. Clinical update enteric fever. BMJ. 2021;372:n437. https://doi.org/10.1136/bmj.n437. Published: 26 February 202 (Remove the numbers following the names of authors)

Saha T, Arisoyin AE, Bollu B, Ashok T, Babu A, Issani A, Jhaveri S, Avanthika C. Enteric fever: diagnostic challenges and the importance of early intervention. Cureus. 2023;15(7):e41831. https://doi.org/10.7759/cureus.41831. PMID: 37575696; PMCID: PMC10423039.

Malaria

7

Contents

> **Key Messages**
> Malaria should be considered in the differential diagnosis of fever of any degree in a child residing in or with a history of travel to an endemic area. *Plasmodium falciparum* infection should be expeditiously treated with a three-day course of artemisinin-based combination therapy (ACT) with close monitoring.

7.1 Case Discussion

A 5-year-old boy was brought with fever and headache for 6 days and with occasional cough and vomiting for 2 days. The maximum temperature noted was 40.2 °C. The fever was accompanied by chills and rigors. He was voiding urine and was active during the afebrile periods. He was a resident of South Chennai, India, and there was a history of recent travel (3 weeks ago) to a village near Cuttack in the state of Odisha for a family function. He received only paracetamol for his fever. There was no history of rash. Other family members were normal. There was no significant illness in the past, and he had received all the vaccines in the Indian Academy of Pediatrics (IAP) schedule till 5 years.

On physical examination, the temperature was 39.5 °C. Otherwise, the general physical examination was normal. There was no lymphadenopathy and oral examination was normal. Abdominal palpation revealed a palpable, soft, nontender liver of 3 cm, and spleen was palpable 2 cm and firm. Liver span was 9 cm. Other systems were normal.

P. Venkat Ramanan, R. Padmanabhan, *Fever in Children*,
https://doi.org/10.1007/978-981-97-9967-1_7

1. *What are the possible causes of this child's short duration fever with hepatosplenomegaly?*

Short duration fever is arbitrarily considered as fever up to 7 days. The causes of such a fever differ in different age groups, geographic locations, and seasons.

The common causes of fever in infants and children in India are viral fever including dengue, acute respiratory infection, acute gastroenteritis, urinary tract infection, rickettsial infections, malaria, and leptospirosis. Rarely mixed infections can occur in children. The presence of hepatosplenomegaly in this child makes undifferentiated viral fevers, acute respiratory infection, and urinary tract infection less likely. Nonspecific respiratory symptoms such as cough and gastrointestinal symptoms can be associated with enteric fever, viral infections including dengue, scrub typhus, or malaria.

2. *What will you do next?*

The child would need to be investigated for the common causes of fever with hepatosplenomegaly: enteric fever, scrub typhus, and malaria. A complete blood count (CBC) along with examination of peripheral smear may help to give some clues regarding the type of infection. Blood culture needs to be sent to rule out enteric fever. Test for dengue such as NS1 antigen is required. Serology-based tests such as IgM ELISA for scrub typhus, leptospirosis, and dengue IgM are preferably sent after 5–7 days of fever. Treatment for enteric fever and scrub typhus may have to be initiated pending blood culture and serology reports.

The child was admitted for evaluation. Laboratory parameters were normal except for a hemoglobin level of 9.8gm/dL (normal 11.5–14.5 g/dL) and slightly elevated liver enzymes (serum aspartate aminotransferase [AST] of 60 units/L (normal: 15–50 units/L) and serum alanine aminotransferase [ALT] of 65 units/L [normal: 5–45 units/L]). Blood culture was sent, and he was put on IV ceftriaxone as empirical treatment for enteric fever. His peripheral blood smear was reported as showing *P. falciparum* ring forms (Fig. 7.1).

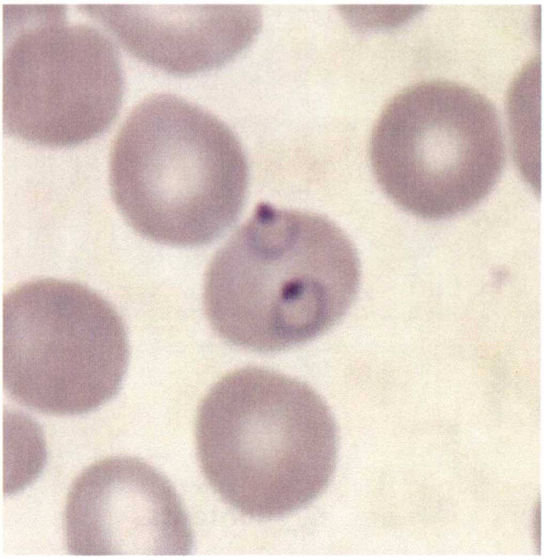

Fig. 7.1 Peripheral smear showing *P. falciparum* ring forms

3. *What are the causative organisms for malaria and their transmission characteristics?*

Malaria is caused by the protozoa *Plasmodium.* There are five species: *P. falciparum*, *P. vivax*, *P. ovale*, *P. malariae*, and the zoonotic *P. knowlesi.* The parasites are transmitted to humans through the bite of infected female *Anopheles* mosquitoes. In sub-Saharan Africa, the vast majority of malaria is due to *P. falciparum*, and in the Asia-Pacific region and the Americas *P. vivax* predominates. *P. falciparum* (*Pf*) malaria is the most severe form of malaria, with fatality rates up to 15% in nonimmune children if appropriate therapy is not promptly instituted. *P. falciparum* infects erythrocytes of all ages and can lead to intense parasitemia which can reach 60% of erythrocytes or more. Malaria caused by other species of plasmodium usually results in parasitemia of less than 2%. *P. vivax* and *P. ovale* preferentially infect reticulocytes, and *P. malariae* infects mostly senescent red cells. Thus, severe complications of malaria are encountered more often in *P. falciparum* infection.

The transmission of malaria depends on the nature of the parasite, the lifespan and feeding habits of the *Anopheles* mosquito, the environment for vector multiplication, and the immune status of the human host. Transmission tends to be more intense with *P. falciparum* and in places where the lifespan of the mosquito is longer and the female *Anopheles* mosquito preferentially bites humans for its blood meal as seen in the African vectors. High-transmission settings include many parts of sub-Saharan Africa and some parts of Oceania. In areas of moderate to high transmission, partial immunity is developed in early childhood, thereby reducing the risk of developing severe malaria in later ages. On the other hand, the low transmission rate of *P. vivax* infection delays acquisition of immunity, so that adults and children alike suffer from acute clinical malaria, with a significant risk for progression to severe malaria if left untreated.

4. *What is the importance of travel history in fever?*

Certain infections are endemic in some regions, and the endemicity may keep changing. Nearly 90% of the world's malaria cases occur in Africa. In the year 2020, globally 241 million cases of malaria were estimated to have occurred with 627,000 deaths. India contributed to 1.7% of malaria cases and 1.2% deaths. In non-endemic areas, malaria occurs mainly in travelers returning from endemic areas. Incidence of malaria has declined in almost all regions of India. States in Southern India such as Kerala and Tamil Nadu are relatively free of malaria. Malaria, mainly of *Plasmodium falciparum* type, is still reported in certain pockets of India. Hence, a history of travel to an area endemic for malaria within or outside the country any time up to 1 year should raise the possibility of malaria in the child presenting with fever.

5. *How does malaria present?*

In endemic areas, malaria should be suspected in any patient presenting with a history of fever and no other obvious cause. The signs and symptoms of malaria are nonspecific and often mimic other common childhood illnesses such as viral fever, gastroenteritis, meningitis/encephalitis, or pneumonia. The clinical manifestations of malaria, severity, and course of malaria depend on the infecting plasmodium species, as well as the age, the ethnicity, malaria-specific immunity, and nutritional status of the child. In areas endemic for malaria, children of less than 5 years of age often get recurrent and severe attacks of the infection. On recovery, they develop partial immunity. Deaths from malaria occur predominantly in children younger than 5 years of age.

The classical pattern of paroxysms of fever on alternate days (tertian fever in *P. vivax*, *P. falciparum*, and *P. ovale infection*) or once every third day (quartan fever in *P. malariae*) is seen in less than 25% of children, and it may take days to evolve. This periodicity requires all the parasites to be developing and getting released from the RBCs into the blood stream simultaneously. It may not occur in asynchronous infections when multiple broods of parasites mature at different periods. *P. falciparum* infections are usually asynchronous, resulting in nonperiodic febrile episodes. The fever may also get modified by the antipyretic treatment. When they occur, the paroxysms are characterized by sudden rise of fever with chills and rigors accompanied by constitutional symptoms such as headache, and exhaustion and spontaneous defervescence in a few hours with profuse sweating. The child may be relatively well in the inter-febrile periods. Respiratory or GI symptoms may be part of malarial infection or may be due to a concomitant infection.

In areas in which malaria transmission is stable (or during the high-transmission period of seasonal malaria), malaria should also be suspected in children with mild fever, anemia, poor appetite, malaise, restlessness, or pallor. Infants and young children more often present with irritability, poor feeding, pallor, lethargy, jaundice, and hepatosplenomegaly along with fever.

On examination, besides fever, pallor may be seen if the infection is prolonged or recurrent. There may be mild hepatomegaly. Splenomegaly may not be seen in the first few days or during the first attack in nonimmune children.

The clinical presentation can be categorized as uncomplicated malaria or severe malaria. Uncomplicated malaria refers to a child with symptoms of malaria and a positive parasitological test but without any feature of end organ damage (severe malaria). When malaria is associated with any of the complications (described later), it is referred to as severe malaria.

In all settings, suspected malaria should be confirmed with a parasitological test, ideally within a short time (<2 h) of the patient presenting. When it is not possible, a decision to provide antimalarial treatment must be based on the probability that the illness is malaria.

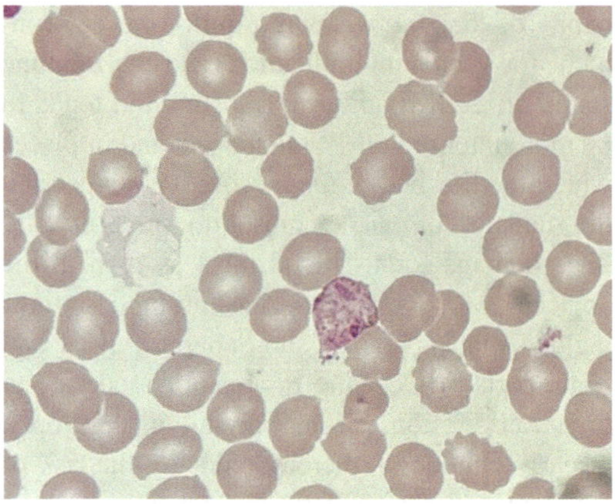

Fig. 7.2 Peripheral smear showing schizont of *P. vivax* Leishman stain 100X

6. *What are the laboratory investigations for malaria?*

The two methods universally used for parasitological diagnosis of malaria are the light microscopy of a peripheral blood smear and immunochromatographic rapid diagnostic tests (RDTs).

Peripheral blood smear examination is considered the gold standard for the diagnosis, and in nearly all cases, the malarial parasite can be identified by a trained microscopist in a thick and thin smear. Blood sample for the test should be collected before the administration of antimalarials. The lowest density for identification by a skilled microscopist is 5–10 parasites/μl blood, but in actual field conditions, it is approximately 100 parasites/μL. A thick film is 10 times more sensitive for diagnosis of malaria and is considered the gold standard; a thin film is useful for species identification (Fig. 7.2) and assessment of the parasite load. It is recommended that examination of 200–500 fields or for 20–30 min is carried out before declaring the smear negative.

Rapid diagnostic tests are to be used when a good quality microscopy is not possible. RDT is based on the detection of parasite-specific antigens or enzymes using monoclonal or polyclonal antibodies. Histidine-rich protein of *P. falciparum* (Pf HRP-2), parasite-specific LDH (pLDH), and pan malarial plasmodium aldolase are the antigens/enzymes targeted. HRP-2 is produced by trophozoites and gametocytes of *P. falciparum*; this antigen persists at detectable levels for >28 days after successful therapy. pLDH is produced by asexual and sexual stages (gametocytes) of all the four plasmodium species.

The advantages of RDT are as follows: (1) no need for electricity/infrastructure, (2) accuracy/ease of use, (3) results can be reported within 15–20 mins, and (4) can be done by a less skilled person. The disadvantages are as follows: (1) cannot quantitate the parasite density, (2) cannot detect the parasite stage, (3) not useful to assess parasite clearance, and (4) high temperature and humidity of tropics may affect the kit. It should be emphasized that negative RDTs do not rule out malaria. Blood smears should be performed to exclude the diagnosis.

Monovalent (Only Pf) and bivalent RDT (Pf and others) kits (Fig. 7.3) are available. Bivalent kits are preferred. If both the slide examination and the RDT are negative, malaria is extremely unlikely, and other causes for the fever should be sought.

Quantitative Buffy Coat (QBC) test is a method for rapid screening of malaria. It uses acridine orange staining and a fluorescent nucleic

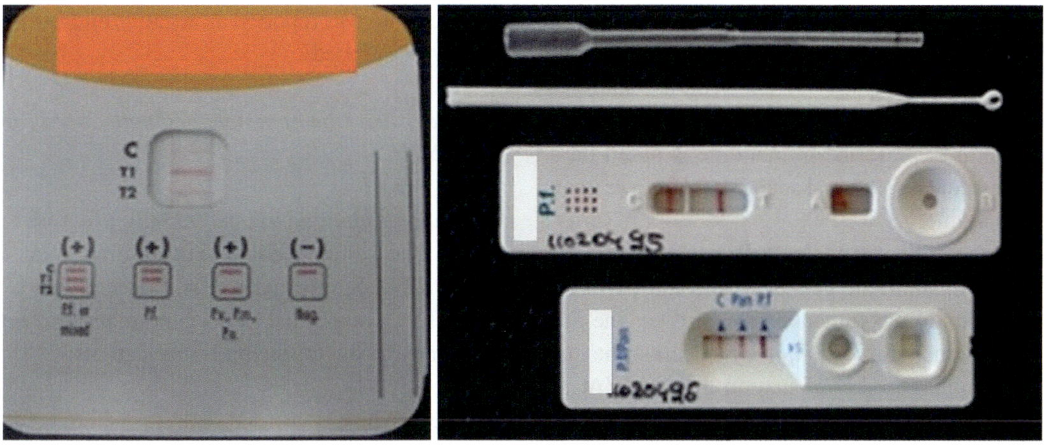

Fig. 7.3 Bivalent RDT kits

acid stain to identify organisms in infected red blood cells. QBC tests are quicker, more sensitive than smear, and easy to perform, but cost is a limiting factor.

Nucleic acid amplification test methods are highly sensitive techniques that are very useful for detecting mixed infections, low parasite densities not detectable by other methods and in drug research. At present, they do not have any role in the clinical management of malaria or in routine surveillance systems.

The WHO strongly advocates a policy of "test, treat, and track" to improve the quality of care and surveillance in malaria.

In hospitalized children, besides a thick and thin blood smear, complete blood count (CBC), serum electrolytes, blood glucose, and renal and liver function tests should be done. CBC may reveal mild anemia and thrombocytopenia even in uncomplicated malaria. Testing for glucose-6-phosphate dehydrogenase (G6PD) deficiency is preferable.

7. *How is malaria treated?*

Treatment of malaria depends on the identification of the plasmodium species, knowledge regarding the resistance pattern in the area where the infection was acquired, national guidelines, and whether the malarial illness is categorized as uncomplicated or severe. Children with uncomplicated malaria who do not have vomiting and who maintain normal hydration can be treated with oral antimalarials on an outpatient basis.

Treatment of Uncomplicated Malaria Due to P. vivax, P. ovale, P. malariae, or P. knowlesi

In areas of chloroquine-susceptible malaria, uncomplicated cases of malaria due to *P. vivax*, *P. ovale*, *P. malariae*, or *P. knowlesi are* treated with chloroquine. *P. vivax* resistant to chloroquine has been recognized since the early 1990s, particularly in the regions of Papua New Guinea and Indonesia. Generally, infections acquired in India are presumed to be chloroquine-sensitive but rare case reports of chloroquine-resistant. *P. vivax* has also been documented in India. In areas of chloroquine-resistant malaria, uncomplicated *P. vivax*, *P. ovale*, *P. malariae*, or *P. knowlesi* malaria is treated with artemisinin-based combination therapy (ACT).

Prevention of Relapse in P. vivax or P. ovale Malaria

To prevent relapse in *P. vivax* and *P. ovale* malaria, children aged >6 months are treated with a 14-day course of primaquine (if they do not have G6PD deficiency). In children with G6PD deficiency, primaquine 0.75 mg/kg may be considered once a week for 8 weeks, with close medical supervision for potential primaquine-induced hemolysis. When G6PD status is unknown and G6PD testing is not available, a decision to prescribe primaquine is based on an assessment of the risks and benefits of giving primaquine.

Uncomplicated Malaria Due to P. falciparum

Artemisinins are generally safe and well tolerated and are recommended by WHO as the first-line treatment for *P. falciparum* malaria. The main artemisinin-based combination therapies (ACTs) are artemether–lumefantrine (AL), artesunate–mefloquine (AS-MQ), artesunate– pyronaridine (AS-PY), artesunate plus sulfadoxine–pyrimethamine (AS+SP), and dihydroartemisinin–piperaquine (DHA-PPQ). In India, the recommended ACT is a 3-day course of AS+SP except in the North Eastern region, where it is AL. On the first day of treatment, in addition to an ACT a single 0.25 mg base/kg primaquine dose should be given in *P. falciparum* malaria to kill the mature gametocytes that are responsible for transmission.

Treating Severe Malaria

Maintaining airway, breathing, and circulation, and monitoring and maintaining blood sugar and serum electrolyte levels are a priority in sick children. Children with severe malaria are treated with intravenous or intramuscular artesunate for at least 24 h or until they can tolerate oral medication, after which the treatment is completed with a 3-day course of ACT. If artesunate is not available, intramuscular artemether is preferred to quinine for treating severe malaria. Though quinine and quinidine can also be used for parenteral treatment of severe malaria, artemisinin is preferred in view of significant mortality reduction compared to the quinine group.

The child was able to take oral medications and hence was started on oral artemisinin-based combination therapy (ACT) of artesunate with sulfadoxine and pyrimethamine. He was monitored round the clock with periodic blood sugar checks. Blood sugar, serum electrolytes, and renal function tests were normal. Later, the blood culture was reported as negative and antibiotics were stopped.

8. *What are the possible complications in children?*

P. falciparum malaria can rapidly progress to severe illness often leading to death if not treated within 24 h. Severe malaria is characterized by the presence of asexual forms in peripheral smear PLUS any of the following complications:

- Altered consciousness with or without seizures (cerebral malaria).
- Respiratory distress or acute respiratory distress syndrome (ARDS).
- Circulatory collapse.
- Metabolic acidosis.
- Renal failure, hemoglobinuria ("blackwater fever").
- Hepatic failure.
- Coagulopathy with or without disseminated intravascular coagulation (DIC).
- Severe anemia or massive intravascular hemolysis.
- Hypoglycemia.

Cerebral malaria can progress rapidly to coma and death and is almost universally fatal if untreated; with treatment, mortality is 15–20%.

P. vivax also is rarely implicated in complicated malaria and multi-organ dysfunction. Repeated attacks of malaria due to *P. vivax* can lead to chronic anemia, malnutrition, and stunted growth.

7.2 Conclusion

The child responded well to a 3-day course of ACT and became afebrile by day 2. A single dose of primaquine also was given on the first day. He was closely monitored and discharged after 3 days with a diagnosis of uncomplicated falciparum malaria. On review after 7 days, he was doing well with regression of liver and spleen. His peripheral smear did not reveal any parasite.

Learning Points

1. Malaria should be considered in any child presenting with any degree of fever in an endemic area or in one who has recently returned from an endemic area.
2. The typical intermittent tertian or quartan fever is not seen commonly in children.
3. Similarly, the paroxysms of fever with chills and rigors may not always be seen.
4. The fever can be associated with respiratory or GI symptoms.
5. Pallor and splenomegaly may not be seen in all the children, especially in the first few days or the first attack.
6. Parasitological diagnosis is done by peripheral smear (PS) examination by light microscopy or rapid diagnostic immunochromatographic kit; PS examination is considered the gold standard.
7. Treatment is based on parasite species and the clinical presentation of uncomplicated or severe malaria.
8. Uncomplicated chloroquine-sensitive *P. vivax* malaria is treated with chloroquine followed by primaquine. Uncomplicated *P. falciparum* malaria is treated with a 3-day course of artemisinin-based combination therapy (ACT).
9. Severe malaria may present with altered sensorium and seizures (cerebral malaria), respiratory distress, severe anemia, hypoglycemia, or any other organ dysfunction.
10. Severe malaria is treated initially with parenteral artemisinin followed by complete course of oral ACT.

Suggested Readings

https://www.who.int/teams/global-malaria-programme/reports/world-malaria-report-2021. Downloaded 4 May 2024.

Schumacher RF, Spinelli E. Malaria in children. Mediterr J Hematol Infect Dis. 2012;4(1):e2012073. https://doi.org/10.4084/MJHID.2012.073. Epub 2012 Nov 6. PMID: 23205261; PMCID: PMC3507524.

WHO guidelines for malaria. WHO-UCN-GMP-2023.01-eng.pdf. Downloaded 10 May 2024.

Parang N Mehta. Pediatric Malaria. Medscape Updated: Jun 03, 2020. https://emedicine.medscape.com/article/998942. Downloaded 3 May 2024.

Hand, Foot, and Mouth Disease with Aseptic Meningitis

8

Contents

> **Key Messages**
> Hand, foot, and mouth disease is common in young children, and aseptic meningitis is a rare complication of the viruses causing HFMD such as Enterovirus 71 (EV71). Simple febrile seizure is a diagnosis of exclusion, and meningitis should always be ruled out when seizures occur in a child 24 h after the onset of fever.

8.1 Case Discussion

A 13-month-old boy, previously well, developmentally normal child, was brought to the ER with a history of fever for 2 days and a generalized tonic-clonic seizures 30 min ago. There was no preceding history of respiratory/gastrointestinal symptoms. He had been fully immunized according to the national immunization schedule, he was the only child, there was no family history of seizures, both parents were working, and the child was in daycare for 8 h/day.

By the time he reached the ER, he had stopped convulsing and was crying but consolable. His sensorium was normal. A general physical examination revealed a well-nourished child. His body temperature was 104.4 °F, with proportionate tachycardia and tachypnea without respiratory distress, a flat anterior fontanelle, and a normal capillary refill time. Meningeal signs could not be elicited as he was crying. There were no rashes and systemic examination was normal. He was started on antipyretic (paracetamol) and IV antibiotic (ceftriaxone) pending CSF examination.

1. *What is the differential diagnosis in a child with fever and seizures and what should be the next step?*

"Febrile seizures" is the term used to describe seizures in a febrile child between 6 months and 5 years of age without evidence of intracranial infection or a defined cause. The peak occurrence of febrile seizures is in children 9–18 months of age. In children younger than 18 months, meningeal signs are not reliable and CSF analysis is recommended whenever there is any doubt. The

P. Venkat Ramanan, R. Padmanabhan, *Fever in Children*,
https://doi.org/10.1007/978-981-97-9967-1_8

absence of any remarkable finding on the history or physical examination and the history of immunization with Hib and pneumococcal conjugate vaccines make bacterial meningitis less likely. Neuroimaging is indicated in a child with fever and seizures with altered sensorium, localizing signs, history of trauma, and associated with neurological findings (developmental delay, microcephaly, or spasticity). MRI is the preferred modality and should be done before lumbar puncture. It requires the child to lie still for over 30 min and is often challenging to perform in acute care settings. Even in simple febrile seizures, the cause of fever needs evaluation as in any other child with fever, and around 2% of infants and children older than 3 months with a temperature above 102.2 °F (39 ° C) are found to have bacteremia. The evaluation of fever in children has been discussed in detail in Chap. 2. In this child, the seizure has occurred 24 h after the onset of fever and there is no past or family history of febrile seizures. Hence, it is mandatory to rule out intracranial infection.

He was hospitalized for evaluation, blood tests were sent, and lumbar puncture was done after fundus evaluation. The laboratory findings revealed normal hemoglobin and platelet count, a WBC count of 7200/cu mm, with 66% polymorphs, a procalcitonin (PCT) level of 0.52 ng/dL, and a CRP value of 1.2 mg/dL. On lumbar puncture, the CSF was clear and the opening pressure was normal. The CSF cell count was reported as 137 WBCs/cu mm with 52% lymphocytes. The CSF cell count suggested meningitis.

2. *What are the causes of meningitis in this age group?*

Meningitis in this age group can be due to infectious (bacterial, viral, rickettsial) as well as noninfectious causes. Among the bacterial causes in infants 3 months to 3 years of age, *Streptococcus pneumoniae* and *Neisseria meningitidis* are the common organisms in this post Hib vaccine era. Enteroviruses (EVs) are the most common cause of viral meningitis followed by herpesviruses, arboviruses, rabies, and influenza. Children with meningitis should be initially presumed to have bacterial meningitis and should be managed accordingly until bacterial meningitis has been excluded (or at least deemed very unlikely) or a specific viral etiology has been identified. Some noninfectious causes include Kawasaki disease, acute demyelinating meningoencephalitis, and drugs like intravenous immunoglobulin and nonsteroidal anti-inflammatory drugs.

In this child, the possibilities of bacterial as well as aseptic meningitis were considered. The CSF was sent for biochemical analysis and culture. IV antibiotic was continued. The CSF biochemistry was reported as glucose of 50 mg/dL with corresponding blood sugar being 92 mg/dL. CSF protein level was 72 mg/dL, and brain magnetic resonance imaging (MRI) was normal.

3. *How can we differentiate between bacterial and viral meningitis?*

The clinical manifestations of viral meningitis are generally similar to those of bacterial meningitis but often are less severe. The clinical clues to a viral etiology include rash, herpangina, conjunctivitis, pharyngitis, pleurodynia, and myopericarditis.

In viral meningitis, the initial CSF white blood cell count typically ranges from 10 to 500 cells/μL. Normal cell counts may be seen in EV and parechovirus infections and rarely in herpes simplex virus (HSV) meningoencephalitis early in the course of infection. There is a predominance of mononuclear cells in most cases of viral meningitis, although a polymorphonuclear neutrophil (PMN) predominance may be seen in the first 24–48 h in EV meningitis. The CSF glucose level is usually ≥40% of the serum value except in mumps meningoencephalitis, in which CSF glucose may be low. CSF protein level is normal to slightly elevated but usually <100 mg/dL. In **bacterial meningitis,** the CSF cell count is usually >1000 cells/μL with a predominance of PMN cells, glucose is <40 mg/dL, and protein is between 100 and 500 mg/dL. Multiplex polymerase chain reaction and gram stain can identify the pathogen.

On day 3 of fever, the child was noted to have rashes in the soles (Fig. 8.1) and this spread to

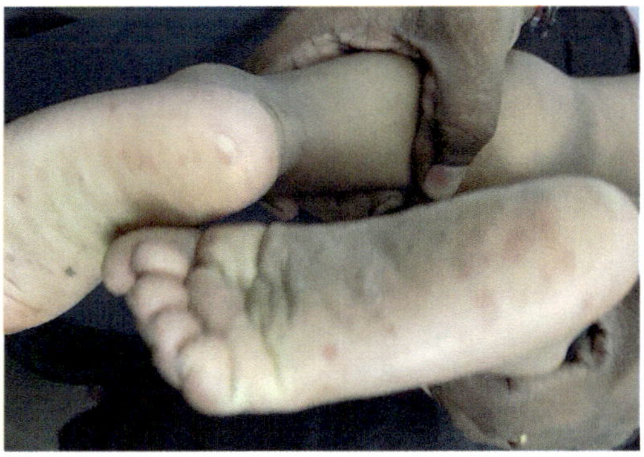

Fig. 8.1 Maculopapular rash with a few vesicles. Photo courtesy Dr. Dhanaratnamoorthy

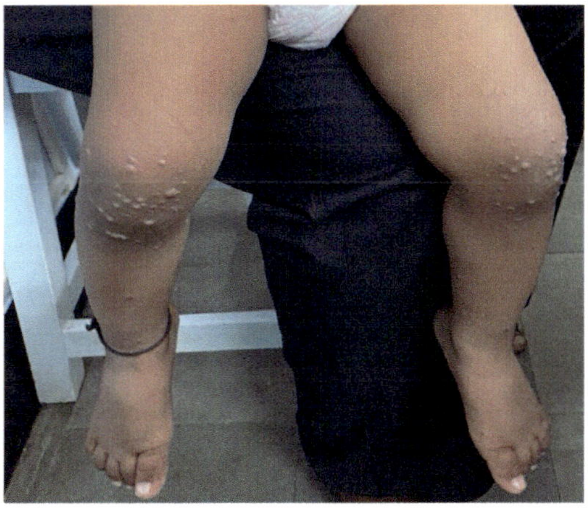

Fig. 8.2 Vesicular rash over both knees. Photo courtesy Dr. Dhanaratnamoorthy

involve the knees and buttocks over the next 2 days (Fig. 8.2). He was also found to have painful blisters on the gums and tongue.

A diagnosis of hand, foot, and mouth disease (HFMD) with aseptic meningitis was made.

4. *What is a hand-foot-mouth disease (HFMD) and how is it acquired?*

HFMD is a viral infection common in young children, caused by several serotypes of enteroviruses with coxsackievirus A16 (CV-A16) being the most common. Enterovirus 71 (EV-71) has been reported to cause outbreaks in Southeast Asia. These viruses are transmitted from person to person by the fecal-oral route, by contact with oral and respiratory secretions, and by the vesicle fluid. The incubation period for HFMD typically is 3–5 days but the range is 2–7 days. The clinical features of HFMD include an abrupt onset of moderate to high fever that is short-lasting, followed in 48 h by painful oral ulcers, refusal to eat (due to pain), and a papulovesicular rash involving the hands, feet, and buttocks.

5. *What are the complications of HFMD?*

Common complications of HFMD may include decreased oral intake due to the painful lesions, which may result in dehydration and may necessitate hospitalization for parenteral fluid therapy. Onychomadesis (shedding of the nail) is a late complication (occurring 3–8 weeks after illness onset), particularly in patients with atypical HFMD (e.g., caused by coxsackievirus A6). Other complications include Gianotti–Crosti syndrome-like eruptions, eczema coxsackium, petechial/purpuric eruption, and vesiculobullous exanthem.

Serious complications rarely occur, except with HFMD caused by EV-71 which has been associated with central nervous system (CNS) disease (brain stem encephalitis, acute flaccid paralysis, aseptic meningitis), myocarditis, pulmonary hemorrhage, edema, and even death. Brain stem encephalitis caused by EV-71 is characterized by myoclonus, ataxia, oculomotor palsies, nystagmus, and bulbar palsy. The most common symptoms are myoclonic jerks and ataxia. Myoclonus may often be overlooked as a benign symptom of febrile illnesses in children. These myclonic jerks occur when the child is awake as well as during light and deep sleep.

6. *How is the diagnosis of HFMD confirmed?*

The diagnosis of HFMD usually is made clinically, based on the typical appearance and location of the oral ulcers and rashes. Identification or isolation of the virus from the throat, vesicular fluid, stool, or cerebrospinal fluid (if HFMD is complicated by meningitis) by PCR confirms the viral etiology. In EV-71 CNS involvement, the MR images may be normal but the characteristic findings in brain stem encephalitis are high signal intensities on T2-weighted images in the posterior pons, medulla oblongata, midbrain, and bilateral dentate nuclei of the cerebellum.

7. *What is the treatment for HFMD*?

Pain and discomfort due to fever can be managed with paracetamol or ibuprofen. Children who are unable to consume enough orally to maintain hydration should be hospitalized for parenteral fluid therapy. Dehydration is corrected with intravenous fluids. Routine use of topical therapies containing lidocaine to coat oral lesions and/or soothe is not recommended. There is no specific antiviral therapy available. Intravenous immunoglobulin (IVIG) therapy has been tried in the management of EV-71 CNS infection. IVIG helps by providing neutralizing antibodies, decreasing sympathetic outflow, and reducing cytokine production. Intravenous milrinone has also been found to be useful in brain stem encephalitis. It has vasodilator and anti-inflammatory properties.

8. *How can enteroviral infections be prevented?*

Hand hygiene is important, and the surfaces and fomites contaminated with oral secretions or feces should be cleaned and disinfected. Strict adherence to hand hygiene protocols is important when changing diapers because EVs are shed in the stool for weeks following infection. Children with active lesions should avoid swimming pools. The viruses that cause HFMD can be spread by children without symptoms and by those whose symptoms have resolved. Hence, the exclusion of symptomatic children from daycare alone may not control the spread.

8.2 Conclusion

Antibiotics were stopped when the culture reports came out negative. Painful oral lesions necessitated parenteral fluid administration for 48 h to maintain hydration. The fever subsided on day 5 of illness. There were no neurological sequelae. The child was discharged and on review, the lesions had resolved.

Learning Points

1. In children younger than 18 months presenting with fever and seizures, meningeal signs are not reliable to exclude meningitis and CSF analysis is recommended whenever there is any doubt.
2. Enteroviruses (EVs) are the most common cause of viral meningitis in children.
3. HFMD is a viral infection common in young children, caused by several serotypes of enteroviruses.
4. The viruses that cause HFMD are transmitted from person to person by the fecal-oral route, by contact with oral and respiratory secretions, and by the vesicle fluid.
5. The diagnosis of HFMD usually is made clinically, based on the typical appearance and location of the oral ulcers and vesicular rashes typically over hands, feet, knees, elbows, and buttocks.
6. Serious complications rarely occur, except with HFMD caused by enterovirus 71 which has been associated with central nervous system disease.
7. All patients with HFMD suspected to be due to EV-71 infection should be carefully observed for headache, vomiting, excessive drowsiness, myoclonus, and ataxia that are early features of CNS involvement.
8. Hand hygiene and disinfection of the contaminated surfaces and fomites are important for preventing infection.

Suggested Readings

Chan KP, Goh KT, Chong CY, Teo ES, Lau G, Ling AE. Epidemic hand, foot and mouth disease caused by human enterovirus 71, Singapore. Emerg Infect Dis. 2003;9(1):78–85.

Gao L, Zou G, Liao Q, et al. Spectrum of enterovirus serotypes causing uncomplicated hand, foot, and mouth disease and enteroviral diagnostic yield of different clinical samples. Clin Infect Dis. 2018;67:1729.

https://iapindia.org/pdf/Ch-060-stg-hand-foot-and-mouth-disease.pdf. Accessed 16 Jul 2024.

Lee KY. Enterovirus 71 infection and neurological complications. Korean J Pediatr. 2016;59(10):395–401. https://doi.org/10.3345/kjp.2016.59.10.395. Epub 2016 Oct 17. PMID: 27826325; PMCID: PMC5099286.

Part II

Fever > 7 Days

Tuberculosis

9

Contents

Key Messages
Tuberculosis is a frequent cause of FUO in adolescents, and miliary pulmonary tuberculosis can present without cough or any respiratory symptoms or signs.

9.1 Case Discussion

A 14-year-old boy, previously well, presented with a history of 12 days of fever, malaise, and fatiguability. There were no localizing symptoms. He had been immunized according to the national immunization schedule till 10 years of age. He had consulted a community physician on day 4 of the illness. A blood test was recommended, and the following reports were available with the parents: Hb 8.4 g/dL, total leucocyte count 4800/cu mm (P 46 L 48 M 2 E 4), platelet count 2.3 lakhs/cu mm, ESR 44 mm first hour, and Widal test: TO 1:40/TH 1:80/AH 1:40/BH 1:40.

The father was told that the child had "typhoid fever" and had been prescribed a course of oral cefixime for 7 days. As there was no change in the fever pattern, he was brought to us. He also gave a history of weight loss, which was however not quantified. There was no history of contact with a case of tuberculosis. There was no history of cough.

1. *Your comment on the Widal test report?*

The traditional Widal test measures antibodies against flagellar (H) and somatic (O) antigens of the causative organisms of enteric fever, i.e., *Salmonella* Typhi and Paratyphi A and B. In acute infection, O antibody appears first, around the end of the first week and rises progressively. H antibody appears a little later but persists longer. Hence, this test should never be recommended in the first week of fever. The Widal test has many limitations. Many small local laboratories offer Widal testing with little quality control. Besides, reliability is less if a slide test is done as compared to a tube test. Raised antibodies may

P. Venkat Ramanan, R. Padmanabhan, *Fever in Children*,
https://doi.org/10.1007/978-981-97-9967-1_9

be due to previous typhoid immunization or earlier infection(s). Many of the antigens targeted for testing are shared among different *Salmonella* serovars. There are no universal standards that define the cut-off dilution of agglutinating antibodies to indicate a positive Widal test, and in endemic countries, where the population has higher titers, 1:160 is taken as the cut-off to suggest enteric fever. For Widal test to be considered confirmatory, a fourfold rise in titer should be demonstrated in paired sera, once during the acute phase and the other during the convalescent phase of the infection, which can be approximately 10–14 days apart. This will not be practicable in the clinical situation. Because of the low specificity of the assay (50–70%) and the inability to differentiate an active infection from previous infection or typhoid vaccination (this is unlikely with the currently available typhoid vaccines), the test is not clinically useful.

On examination, he was pale and thin with a weight of 40 kg and a BMI of <third centile. BCG scar was present. The axillary temperature recorded was 102.1 °F. The pulse rate was 92/min and the respiratory rate was 18/min. He was ill-appearing and his hydration was normal. There was no hepatosplenomegaly or lymph node enlargement. General physical (including skin for rash, eschar) and systemic examinations were also normal. A dilated funduscopic examination was normal.

2. *What would be your differential diagnosis and further management?*

The term "fever of unknown origin" (FUO) is used in children with fever >38.3 °C (101 °F) for at least 8 days' duration, in whom no diagnosis is apparent after initial clinical evaluation and initial laboratory assessment. The common etiologies fall under three categories: infections, connective tissue diseases, and malignancies, and the causes vary according to the geographical region, age group, and immune status of the patient. In children, FUO is usually caused by common infections, with an unusual presentation and evaluation is best done after hospitalization.

The child was hospitalized. A complete blood count revealed normocytic normochromic anemia, but the total and differential counts and platelet counts were normal. An antinuclear antibody (ANA) screening test was done for systemic lupus erythematosus (SLE), and the result was negative. Peripheral blood smear showed no abnormal cells or hemoparasites. ESR was 74 mm in the first hour. LFT and RFT were normal. Blood and urine cultures showed no growth. Chest X-ray (Fig. 9.1), echocardiography, and ultrasound of the abdomen were normal. The Mantoux test was negative.

Throughout hospitalization, he was noted to have fever with a maximum temperature of 103.4 °F. Daily examination revealed no new clinical clues.

3. *What would you do next?*

In the evaluation of FUO, the first tier of investigations are complete blood count, LFT and RFT, three or more blood cultures, erythrocyte sedimentation rate (ESR), C-reactive protein (CRP), human immunodeficiency virus (HIV) serology, peripheral blood smears for malarial parasites, urine analysis and culture, chest X-ray, abdominal ultrasound, sputum smears for acid-

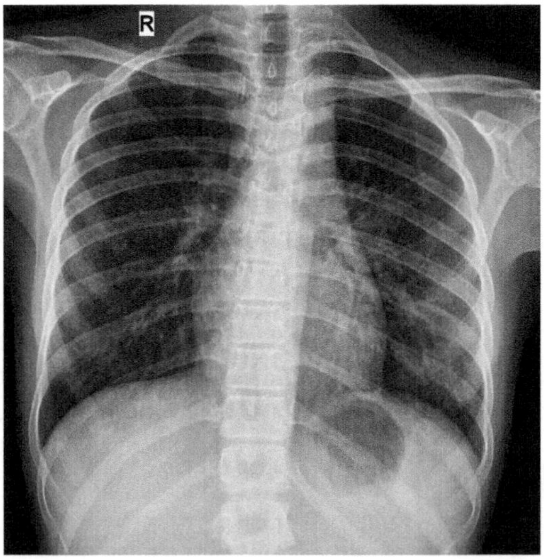

Fig. 9.1 Normal chest X-ray. (Photo courtesy Dr. T. Rishab Ramesh)

fast bacilli (AFB) if there is cough, and thyroid function tests. In children less than 5 years, resting gastric juice or induced sputum for identification of *Mycobacterium Tuberculosis* (MTB) by cartridge-based nucleic acid amplification test (CBNAAT) is required. For those who remain undiagnosed, the second-tier tests are echocardiogram, antinuclear antibody (ANA), and CT scans. A bone marrow aspiration/biopsy is considered especially when there are hematological abnormalities, lymphadenopathy, or organomegaly.

In this child, in view of high ESR and history of weight loss, the possibilities of tuberculosis (TB) and malignancies like lymphoma were considered, and CT scans of the thorax and abdomen were done. CT scan of the chest (Fig. 9.2a, b) showed multiple centrilobular nodules of varying sizes in "tree in bud" configuration scattered in both the lungs suggestive of miliary tuberculosis (TB). Some of these nodules were seen coalescing to form small patchy areas of consolidation with surrounding ground glassing.

4. *Can the chest X-ray be normal when there is a significant finding on the chest CT scan?*

In miliary disease, the classic chest X-ray image is a fine reticulonodular infiltrate throughout the lungs. Other abnormalities include pleural reactions, hilar or mediastinal adenopathy, and interstitial infiltrates. The chest X-ray is normal in up to 50% of patients with miliary TB. In some, the changes are subtle and are picked up only by experienced chest radiologists. High-resolution computed tomography (HRCT) of the chest is more sensitive for miliary TB than plain chest radiography.

5. *Can treatment for TB be initiated based on this radiological finding?*

No. These findings are not specific to miliary TB and may also be seen in other infectious (bacteria, fungi, *Mycoplasma pneumoniae*) and non-infectious diseases (sarcoidosis, metastasis, hypersensitivity pneumonitis, and pneumoconiosis). To establish a diagnosis of TB, a *microbiological diagnosis* has to be made by demonstrating *mycobacterium tuberculosis* (MTB) by acid-fast smear, culture, or CBNAAT like GeneXpert MTB/RIF assay in appropriate samples. For MTB culture, commercial liquid-medium automated detection systems like BACTEC and MGIT 960 are faster and more sensitive than standard techniques using solid medium to isolate MTB. When lesions are present in the lungs, the samples examined are sputum or gastric aspirates (if sputum is not available or the smears are negative). Bronchoscopy is warranted if the diagnosis cannot be established after examination of the sputum or gastric aspirate.

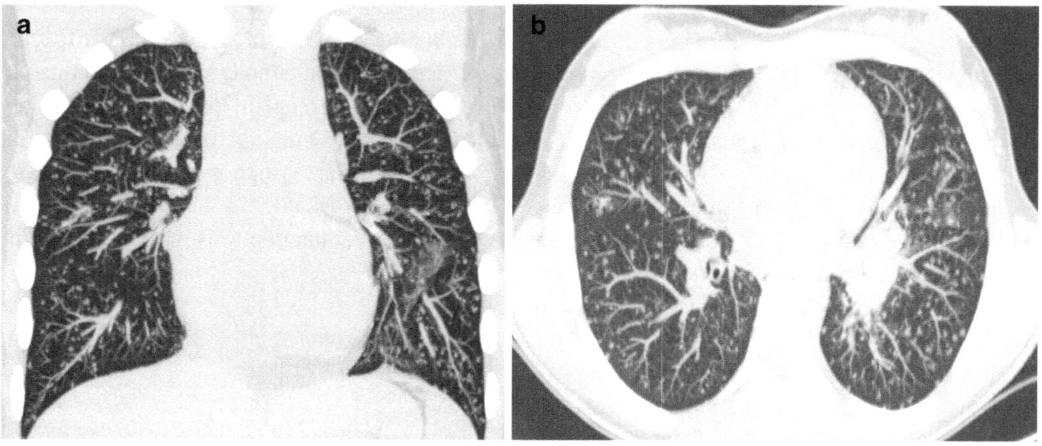

Fig. 9.2 (**a**, **b**) CT scan of the chest showing multiple centrilobular nodules of varying sizes in "tree in bud" configuration scattered in both the lungs. (Photo courtesy Dr. T. Rishab Ramesh)

6. *If the sputum smear is positive for AFB, is it still necessary to send the sample for GeneXpert assay?*

Yes. AFB seen in sputum smear does not give any idea about the drug sensitivity. Hence, Xpert MTB/RIF assay is also done simultaneously. It is a cartridge-based automated nucleic acid amplification test (CBNAAT) that simultaneously identifies *M. tuberculosis* and rifampicin resistance (RR).

7. *Is it necessary to do a sputum culture for AFB in all cases?*

Cultures should be sent in all children who are CBNAAT negative and all presumptive DR TB (RNTCP Updated Pediatric TB Guidelines 2019. Guidance document Developed by Revised National Tuberculosis Control Program and Indian Academy of Pediatrics).

CBNAAT, in addition to detecting MTB, provides information about rifampicin resistance. When rifampicin resistance (RR) is seen, the patient is offered first-line (FL) and second-line (SL) Line Probe Assay (LPA). Direct LPA can be performed only on smear-positive specimens. In instances where the AFB smear is negative, culture is set up, and if the culture is positive, an indirect LPA is performed on the isolate.

The yield of culture can be less than 40%, with slightly higher sensitivity and faster results in liquid mycobacterial growth in tube compared with solid culture media.

8. *How often is it possible to establish a microbiological diagnosis? What are the other tests that can support the diagnosis?*

The sensitivity of sputum smear for acid-fast bacilli is only 35–70%, requiring 5000–10,000 bacteria/mL of sputum. The nucleic acid amplification (NAA) method is quicker and has a higher sensitivity of 60–70%.

Histopathology of tissue biopsy specimens in TB typically demonstrates granulomas composed of epithelioid macrophages, Langhans giant cells, and lymphocytes with central caseation ("cheese-like") necrosis; organisms may or may not be seen with acid-fast staining. In the appropriate clinical and epidemiologic settings, they strongly support a diagnosis of TB, but it is important to try and establish a microbiological diagnosis.

9. *What is miliary tuberculosis and how does it present?*

Miliary tuberculosis (TB) results from the hematogenous dissemination of *Mycobacterium tuberculosis* to the lungs and other organs from progressive primary infection or via reactivation of a latent focus. Miliary TB was seen more commonly in infants, children less than 4 years, and in the immunocompromised. However, currently, the disease is being increasingly reported in adolescents and young adults and in the elderly. It is characterized by small, firm white nodules resembling millet seeds in the organs involved which include the lungs, the lymphatic system, bones and joints, liver, spleen, central nervous system (CNS), and adrenal glands. Acute disease may be fulminant, including multi-organ system failure, a syndrome of septic shock, and acute respiratory distress syndrome (ARDS). Patients with subacute or chronic disease may present with failure to thrive, fever of unknown origin, or dysfunction of one or more organ systems.

The presence of choroid tubercles caused by hematogenous seeding of the choroid, seen on fundoscopy in 5–20% of cases, is one of the few clinical findings with high specificity for disseminated tuberculosis.

Laboratory investigations provide nonspecific evidence of a chronic multi-system inflammatory disorder. Fifty percent of patients with miliary tuberculosis are anemic. Around 80% with miliary tuberculosis are lymphopenic, rising to nearly 100% if the bone marrow has been infiltrated. Abnormal liver function tests are seen when the liver is involved.

10. *Does BCG vaccination protect against disseminated TB?*

Though BCG vaccination protects from disseminated TB like miliary TB, the protective efficacy is controversial ranging from 0% to 80%.

11. *Can the Mantoux test be negative in a child with active TB?*

A positive Mantoux test suggests TB infection (though not an active disease), but a negative result does not rule out TB. False-negative Mantoux is seen more commonly in miliary TB than in pulmonary or isolated extrapulmonary TB and is reported to be as high as 68%.

In miliary tuberculosis, transbronchial lung biopsy may demonstrate granulomatous inflammatory lesions up to 60%.

12. *What is the role of steroids in the treatment of miliary TB?*

The only definite indications for steroids in miliary TB are TB involving the CNS or the pericardium.

9.2 Conclusion

In this child, sputum and gastric aspirate were negative for AFB. A bronchoscopy was done, and the bronchoalveolar lavage smear was positive for AFB; by GeneXpert MTB was detected, and RIF resistance was not detected. On contact survey, no other case was detected in the family.

As per the protocol, HIV testing was done which was found to be negative. The child was treated with the traditional regimen category 1 for 6 months and he recovered completely.

Learning Points

1. Tuberculosis is a frequent cause of FUO in adolescents, even among the immunocompetent.
2. Clinical features of tuberculosis are non-specific, and patients with miliary pulmonary tuberculosis can present without any respiratory signs on examination.
3. Miliary TB is reported increasingly more frequently in older children and adolescents.
4. Chest X-ray may be normal in 50% of individuals with miliary pulmonary TB, and the diagnosis is made only by a chest CT scan.
5. Every attempt to establish a microbiological diagnosis from appropriate samples should be made.
6. Molecular tests like GeneXpert are useful rapid diagnostic tools.
7. The approach to antimicrobial therapy for treatment of miliary TB is the same as for pulmonary TB using a traditional multidrug regimen (≥6 months); modifications may be warranted in the setting of drug-resistant TB.
8. A negative Mantoux test does not rule out TB.

Suggested Readings

https://iapindia.org/pdf/Ch-149-Diagnosis-and-Management-of-Childhood-Tuberculosis.pdf.

National Tuberculosis Elimination Programme. Paediatric TB management guideline. 2022. https://tbcindia.gov.in/showfile.php?lid=3668. Accessed 9 Jul 2024.

Vohra S, Dhaliwal HS. Miliary tuberculosis. In: StatPearls. Treasure Island, FL: StatPearls Publishing; 2024.

World Health Organization. Guidance for national tuberculosis programmes on the management of tuberculosis in children. https://apps.who.int/iris/bitstream/handle/10665/112360/9789241548748_eng.pdf?sequence=1. Accessed 9 Jul 2024.

Brucellosis 10

Contents

> **Key Messages**
> Brucellosis is a relatively common zoonotic infection and should always be considered in the differential diagnosis of prolonged fever with hepatosplenomegaly. The diagnosis is confirmed by blood or bone marrow culture preferably using automated culture systems like Bactec and BacTAlert.

10.1 Case Discussion

An 11-year-old boy presented with a history of moderate-grade remittent fever with chills for 9 days. He had mild abdominal pain with occasional loose stools in the first 3 days. He had consulted a local doctor on day 4 of fever and had been started on oral cefixime for possible enteric fever. The loose stools and abdominal pain subsided but fever persisted. From day 7 of the illness, he also developed backache and joint pains. He had no other respiratory, gastrointestinal, or urinary symptoms. There was no significant past medical or surgical history. He was immunized according to the national immunization schedule. His family members were healthy. They lived in a rural town, but there were no domestic animals at home. He always consumed only home food and boiled milk.

On physical examination, the child was alert. There was no pallor, icterus, skin rashes, or significant lymphadenopathy. Systemic examination revealed a liver of 2 cm and a spleen of 2 cm; both were soft and nontender. The possibilities of enteric fever, scrub typhus, and malaria were considered. He was hospitalized and started on oral doxycycline and intravenous (IV) ceftriaxone, (for scrub typhus and enteric fever respectively), and he was investigated accordingly.

His investigations revealed a hemoglobin level of 10.9 g/dL, a WBC count of 8250 cells/mm^3, with 53% neutrophils, a platelet count of 90,000 lacs/mm^3, and an erythrocyte sedimentation rate (ESR) of 27 mm/h (<15 mm/h). His C-reactive protein (CRP) was normal. Peripheral smear did not reveal any hemoparasites or abnormal cells. The serum aspartate aminotransferase (AST) was 65 U/L

P. Venkat Ramanan, R. Padmanabhan, *Fever in Children*,
https://doi.org/10.1007/978-981-97-9967-1_10

(0–35 U/L), alanine aminotransferase (ALT) was 57 U/L (0–45 U/L), and albumin was 4.1 mg/dL (3.2–4.5 mg/dL). Renal function tests and serum bilirubin were normal.

Serology for scrub typhus was negative. Oral doxycycline was stopped. After 48 h, the blood and urine cultures were negative. Radiologic examination of the lungs, heart, and abdomen was normal. An abdominal ultrasound showed enlarged liver and spleen. The fever continued unabated.

1. *What are the differential diagnoses to be considered on day 12 for fever with hepatosplenomegaly, thrombocytopenia, and mildly elevated liver enzymes?*

With the above clinical features and laboratory investigations, the differential diagnosis has to be considered under three main categories: infections, autoimmune conditions, and malignancies.

Among infections, enteric fever, scrub typhus (negative in this child), infective endocarditis (IE), Epstein–Barr virus (EBV), and disseminated TB are the more likely ones in South India. The blood culture may be sterile due to the prior use of antibiotics. Infection associated with hemophagocytic lymphohistiocytosis (HLH) can also cause cytopenia with persistent fever. Autoimmune diseases such as systemic lupus erythematosus (SLE) and systemic juvenile idiopathic arthritis (SJIA) may present like this though the TLC and platelet count are more likely to be raised in SJIA. Hematological malignancies like leukemia also need to be considered. Repeated clinical examination for fresh clues and repeat investigations will be needed to uncover the cause.

The child was re-examined, and there were no new clinical findings apart from a few cervical and axillary lymph nodes 0.5–1 cm in size. Repeat CBC revealed a Hb level of 9.2 g/dL with normal TC/DC and a platelet count of 67,000/cu mm. The Mantoux test was nonreactive, and serology test results for cytomegalovirus (CMV), HIV, EBV, and hepatitis A, B, and C viruses were negative. Repeat peripheral blood smear revealed pancytopenia but no abnormal or malignant cells. An abdominal CT scan showed hepatosplenomegaly and a few mesenteric lymph nodes with mild ascites. Echocardiography did not show pericardial effusion or vegetation. A bone marrow examination was planned.

2. *What are the indications for a bone marrow tap in the evaluation of pyrexia of unknown origin (PUO) in children?*

Bone marrow examination is useful in uncovering the cause of PUO where initial investigations have not yielded a diagnosis. It is more likely to contribute to the diagnosis when there are hematological abnormalities like cytopenia in the peripheral blood. It helps in identifying infections like tuberculosis, visceral leishmaniasis, CMV, and fungal infections. Bone marrow culture is less affected by prior antibiotic use and is often positive in infections like enteric fever and staph sepsis. Malignancies like lymphomas with marrow involvement and leukemias can be diagnosed by bone marrow examination. Conditions like sarcoidosis and systemic lupus erythematosus can sometimes be recognized by the characteristic findings in the marrow.

Bone marrow aspiration showed normocellular marrow with normal erythropoiesis and granulopoiesis with no maturation abnormality or hemoparasites. The bone marrow culture was processed by an automated BacT/Alert system. On the fourth day of incubation, the system gave a positive beep. Gram stain from the positive culture bottle showed small gram-negative coccobacilli. A diagnosis of probable brucellosis was made. Ceftriaxone was stopped, and treatment with doxycycline and rifampicin was initiated. On further probing, the boy revealed that one of his friends had a goat farm and he would often play with goats and pet them.

3. *What is brucellosis and what are its clinical features?*

Brucellosis is a systemic infection caused by *Brucellae*, which are small gram-negative coccobacilli. It is the most common zoonotic infection globally and affects all age groups, particularly in resource-limited settings. It is also known as "undulant fever," "Mediterranean fever," or "Malta fever." Four *Brucella* species can affect humans: *B. melitensis* (from sheep, goats, and camels), *B. abortus* (from cattle), *B. suis* (from swine), and *B. canis* (from dogs). *B. melitensis* is the most common among these. The clinical features of brucellosis are variable and nonspecific. It typically causes fever of insidious onset, malaise, night sweats, fatigue, weakness, backache, and arthralgias. The characteristic fever pattern is daily spikes with chills and night sweats and can persist for weeks if untreated. Hence the term "undulant fever." On examination, there may be hepatomegaly, splenomegaly, and/or lymphadenopathy.

4. *How do children acquire the infection?*

Brucellosis is usually acquired from infected animals by consumption of food products (such as unpasteurized milk and milk products). The bacteria can survive for weeks in dairy products but are killed by boiling, pasteurization, and fermentation. Transmission can also occur by contact of skin or mucous membranes with infected animal tissue fluids (such as placenta, blood, urine, or milk) or inhalation of infected aerosolized particles. After entering the body, the organism is taken up by local tissue lymphocytes. They multiply in the lymph nodes from where they enter the circulation and seed throughout the body. The incubation period is usually 5–60 days but may be as long as several months.

The coccobacillus was identified as *Brucella melitensis by matrix-assisted laser desorption ionization–time of flight mass spectrometry (MALDI-TOF MS)*. The diagnosis of brucellosis was confirmed. The initial treatment was continued. Fever subsided after 8 days of treatment after which he was discharged and advised to continue the therapy at home for a total duration of 6 weeks.

5. *How is brucellosis diagnosed?*

A definitive diagnosis is made by culture of the organism from blood, body fluids (urine, cerebrospinal fluid, synovial fluid, or pleural fluid), or tissue (such as bone marrow or liver biopsy). Automated cultures and *MALDI-TOF MS are useful for rapid identification of microbes with high sensitivity.*

A fourfold or greater rise in *Brucella* antibody titer between acute and convalescent-phase serum specimens obtained ≥2 weeks apart is also diagnostic, but this is not useful for initiating therapy. Bone marrow culture is more sensitive, has a shorter time to detection than blood culture, and its sensitivity is not diminished by prior antibiotic use.

A presumptive diagnosis of brucellosis can be made when the *Brucella* antibody titer is ≥1:160 by standard tube agglutination test (SAT) or when *Brucella* DNA is detected in a clinical specimen by polymerase chain reaction (PCR) assay. High-resolution molecular methods (singleplex and multiplex PCR) have been developed for *Brucella* spp. identification. Rapid genus-level and species-level identification is possible via 16S rRNA (ribosomal RNA) gene sequencing and real-time PCR-based analysis.

A compatible clinical picture, such as arthralgia, prolonged fever, sweating, chills, headache, and malaise, and exposure to goats/sheep where the symptoms resolve with anti-brucellosis therapy can also be accepted for diagnosis when both cultures and serology are negative.

6. *What are the special precautions in blood culture for brucellosis?*

In laboratories where conventional blood cultures are being done, the laboratory workers should be informed about the diagnostic possibility of brucellosis so that appropriate precautions are taken, special culture techniques are used, and the bottles are incubated for a long time. Subcultures should be performed for at least 4 weeks. The growth of *Brucellae* is detected in 7 and 21 days and the yield is variable (40–90% in acute disease versus 5–20% in chronic, focal, or complicated disease). It requires level 3 biocontainment facilities and trained personnel to handle samples. Nowadays, most microbiology laboratories use automated culture systems like Bactec and BacTAlert. They are safe and fast methods for diagnosis. The organism may be detected as early as day 3 of incubation, and most isolates are recovered in 1 week; the bottles need not be incubated for longer than 2 weeks. Cultures of fluids other than blood or tissues may take up to 3 weeks to grow on plated media. Blood cultures are often negative in chronic disease.

7. *What are the serological tests that are useful in making a diagnosis of brucellosis?*

The most common tests are the standard tube agglutination test (SAT) and enzyme-linked immunosorbent assays (ELISAs). SAT titers >1:160 outside endemic regions and >1:320 within endemic areas are considered positive. A fourfold or greater rise in the titer between acute and convalescent-phase serum specimens obtained ≥2 weeks is also diagnostic but is clinically not useful as it may delay therapy.

Rose Bengal agglutination test and the immunochromatographic lateral flow assay are screening tests. For patients with complicated and/or chronic infection, the 2-mercaptoethanol (2-ME) agglutination test, the immunocapture agglutination (Brucellacapt) test, and the indirect Coombs test are useful. In acute disease, any of the assays may be positive; in chronic disease, non-agglutinating antibodies are more abundant than the agglutinating ones and the SAT may be falsely negative, while 2-ME, Brucellacapt, Coombs, and ELISA IgG may be positive.

Molecular tests are not routinely used but are useful in patients with seronegative tests. Positive molecular test results cannot discriminate between active disease and prior (resolved) brucellar infection. 16S rRNA gene sequencing is useful for genus identification but cannot be used for species identification.

8. *What are the other investigations useful in the management of brucellosis?*

Acute brucellosis may be associated with elevated transaminases and hematologic abnormalities including anemia, leukopenia, or leukocytosis with relative lymphomonocytosis, thrombocytopenia, elevated CRP, and ESR. Bone marrow biopsy may demonstrate non-caseating granulomas. Depending upon the clinical presentation, other investigations may be useful. In joint involvement, the synovial fluid shows elevated white blood cell count usually ≤15,000 cells/μL, which is lymphocyte predominant. The organism can be grown in synovial fluid. In neurologic involvement, CSF shows a cell count of 10–200 predominantly mononuclear cells, mild to moderate elevation of protein levels, low glucose levels, and elevated adenosine deaminase (ADA) levels (may also be observed in the setting of tuberculosis and other infections). The organism is rarely grown in the CSF, but antibody or agglutination testing of the CSF can establish the diagnosis.

9. *How is brucellosis treated?*

For children ≥8 years with brucellosis (without focal involvement like spondylitis, neurobrucellosis, or endocarditis), the preferred regime is oral doxycycline and rifampicin (oral) for 6 weeks. Other options are oral doxycycline for 6 weeks with either IV streptomycin for the first 14–21 days or IV gentamicin for the first 7–10 days.

For children <8 years with uncomplicated brucellosis, the treatment is oral trimethoprim–sulfamethoxazole (TMP-SMX) with rifampicin for 6 weeks. Doxycycline is not recommended for children <8 years of age because of the risk for staining of the teeth.

Relapse is known to occur, and it usually happens within 6 months from completion of treatment. The treatment is with a repeat course of the same regimen.

Children ≥8 years of age with neurobrucellosis are treated with ceftriaxone for the first 4–6 weeks, along with rifampicin and doxycycline, and the duration of therapy is 3–6 months. For children <8 years, TMP-SMX is used in the place of doxycycline.

Brucella endocarditis requires a combination of antimicrobial therapy (an aminoglycoside like streptomycin or gentamicin) for the first month along with rifampicin and doxycycline (for 3–6 months) and early surgery.

10. *How can brucellosis be prevented?*

Currently, there are no vaccines for the prevention of brucellosis in humans. Prevention involves avoiding consumption of raw milk and products made from raw milk and contact of skin or mucous membranes with infected tissue and fluids (such as blood, urine, or milk) of animals. In laboratories, *Brucella* cultures should be performed with biosafety level 3 practices and containment equipment. Vaccines are available against *Brucella abortus* in cattle and against *B. melitensis* in sheep and goats.

11. *What are the complications of brucellosis?*

Complications are not as common in children as in adults. The infection can affect any organ system and cause focal complications. Osteoarticular disease can cause peripheral arthritis, sacroiliitis, and spondylitis. Genitourinary involvement may cause orchitis and/or epididymitis, prostatitis and testicular abscess, tubo-ovarian abscess, cystitis, glomerulonephritis, and renal abscess. Brucellosis in pregnant women increases the risk of spontaneous abortion, fetal death, premature delivery, and intrauterine infection. Neurobrucellosis can manifest as meningitis (acute or chronic), encephalitis, brain abscess, myelitis, radiculitis, and/or neuritis (with involvement of cranial or peripheral nerves). Endocarditis is the most common cardiovascular complication (1–2% of cases) and is the main cause of death attributable to brucellosis. Pulmonary involvement may cause bronchitis, interstitial pneumonitis, lobar pneumonia, lung nodules, pleural effusion, hilar lymphadenopathy, empyema, or abscesses.

Intra-abdominal manifestations include hepatic or splenic abscess, cholecystitis, pancreatitis, ileitis, colitis, and peritonitis. Ocular manifestations include uveitis, keratoconjunctivitis, corneal ulcers, iridocyclitis, nummular keratitis, choroiditis, optic neuritis, papilledema, and endophthalmitis. Dermatologic manifestations include macular, maculopapular, scarlatiniform, papulonodular, and erythema nodosum-like eruptions, ulcerations, petechiae, purpura, granulomatous vasculitis, and abscesses.

12. *What is chronic brucellosis?*

There is no specific definition for chronic brucellosis. Brucellosis is called chronic when clinical manifestations persist for more than one year after the initial diagnosis. There are two categories of chronic brucellosis, those with a focal complication (such as spondylitis, osteomyelitis, tissue abscess, or uveitis) and evidence of infection (positive serology or cultures) and those with persistent symptoms (malaise, depression, anxiety, insomnia, sexual disturbances), tremor, or arthralgias without objective signs of infection.

Relapse following treatment may occur in 5–15%. The cause may be an inadequate antibiotic regimen, inadequate duration of antibiotic therapy, lack of adherence, or localized foci of infection. Relapse usually occurs within the first 6 months following completion of treatment but may occur up to 12 months later. Relapse due to antibiotic resistance is rare.

10.2 Conclusion

The child tolerated the treatment well. By 4 weeks of treatment, he had complete resolution of hepatosplenomegaly and had a normal CBC. He continued to do well on his 6-month follow-up after therapy was completed.

Learning Points

1. Brucellosis is the most common zoonotic disease worldwide.
2. The typical symptoms in children are fever, malaise/myalgia, and arthralgia.
3. The possibility should be considered in the differential diagnosis of prolonged fever in children, especially when there is a history of exposure to cattle, goats, or other farm animals.
4. A high index of suspicion is needed as the clinical and laboratory characteristics can mimic other infectious and noninfectious conditions.

5. Awareness about the myriad manifestations can minimize delays in the diagnosis.
6. Brucellosis in children is frequently mild, self-limited, and less likely to be chronic compared to adults.
7. There is multisystem involvement, and the infection can affect any organ system and cause focal complications, but complications are not as common in children as in adults.
8. The gold standard for diagnosis is the isolation of *Brucella* spp. from samples. Automated culture systems are safer and faster.
9. The laboratory should be informed in advance before sending the sample so that lab personnel may be protected and observation for growth is done for a longer period.
10. A presumptive diagnosis can be made when the *Brucella* antibody titer is $\geq$1:160 by standard tube agglutination test (SAT) or when *Brucella* DNA is detected in a clinical specimen by polymerase chain reaction (PCR) assay.
11. Uncomplicated brucellosis is treated with oral doxycycline or trimethoprim-sulfamethoxazole (TMP-SMX) along with rifampicin for 6 weeks.

Suggested Readings

Centers for Disease Control (CDC). Brucellosis reference guide. 2017. https://www.cdc.gov/brucellosis/pdf/brucellosi-reference-guide.pdf. Accessed 18 Jun 2024.

Dadar M, Shahali Y, Whatmore AM. Human brucellosis caused by raw dairy products: a review on the occurrence, major risk factors and prevention. Int J Food Microbiol. 2019;292:39–47.

Elham E, Bukhari MD. Pediatric brucellosis. An update review for the new millennium. Saudi Med J. 2018;39:336–41.

Kawasaki Disease

11

Contents

> **Key Messages**
> The diagnosis of Kawasaki disease should be considered in any child with unexplained fever for >5 days even when the clinical criteria for typical KD are not met. Early diagnosis and early initiation of IVIG (within 7 days) is important to decrease the complication of coronary aneurysm.

11.1 Case Discussion

A 10-month-old, previously healthy female infant presented with a high-grade fever for 2 days. There were no neurological, respiratory, gastrointestinal, genitourinary, or musculoskeletal symptoms. Clinical examination did not reveal any rashes or focus of infection. In view of high fever, a complete blood count, serum C-reactive protein (CRP) levels, and urine routine were examined. Urine automated microscopy report revealed 10–12 pus cells/HPF though nitrites were absent. Hence urine culture was sent, and she was started on oral antibiotics for possible urinary tract infection (UTI).

She was reviewed after 48 h. High fever persisted, but there were no localizing symptoms or signs. She was also becoming irritable, but there were no signs of meningitis. Other laboratory findings were as follows: white blood cell count (WBC) was 8500/mL (4000–11,000/mL); the differential count was neutrophils (N): 65% (40–75), lymphocytes (L%): 22.8% (40–60), and hemoglobin (Hb): 10 (11–15) g/dL; platelet (PLT) count was 2.4 lacs/mL (1–3 lacs/mL); C-reactive protein (CRP) level was 1.3 (<0.8) mg/dL; and erythrocyte sedimentation rate (ESR) was 40 (0–15) mm/first hour. Urine culture showed no growth.

1. *What are the causes of sterile pyuria?*

Pus cells can be present in sterile urine in several infectious and noninfectious conditions. The infectious causes include viral, tuberculous, fungal, and parasitic infection, and bacterial urinary infections with recent antibiotic therapy. The

P. Venkat Ramanan, R. Padmanabhan, *Fever in Children*,
https://doi.org/10.1007/978-981-97-9967-1_11

noninfectious causes include systemic diseases like vasculitis, renal diseases like glomerulonephritis, drug related, and inflammation adjacent to the genitourinary tract. Hence, the clinician should consider the clinical context in the differential diagnosis.

In view of the irritability and high CRP, a diagnosis of possible sepsis was made. She was hospitalized, blood culture was sent, and oral cefixime was changed to intravenous ceftriaxone. Even after 48 h of hospitalization and IV antibiotics, fever and irritability persisted. No bacterial growth was detected in any of her cultures. Abdominal ultrasonography and chest radiograph were normal.

2. *What are the possible causes of fever not responding to parenteral antibiotics?*

Response to antibiotics is seen only when the cause of fever is a bacterial infection, and the bacteria are susceptible to the antibiotic selected. In this child, though there was pyuria, the absence of nitrites in the urine makes UTI less likely and the urine culture was also sterile. Hence, the possibility of other occult infections and noninfectious causes have to be considered. The child must be re-examined for new signs that might have appeared, and investigations will have to be repeated.

On re-examination (day 6 of illness), bilateral subtle conjunctival injection (Fig. 11.1) was

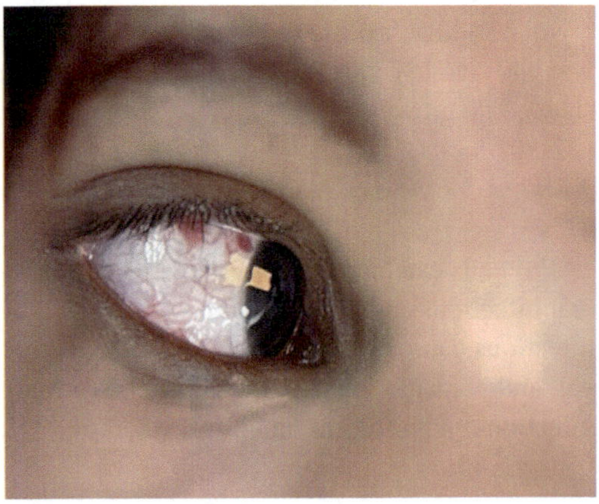

Fig. 11.1 Conjunctival injection

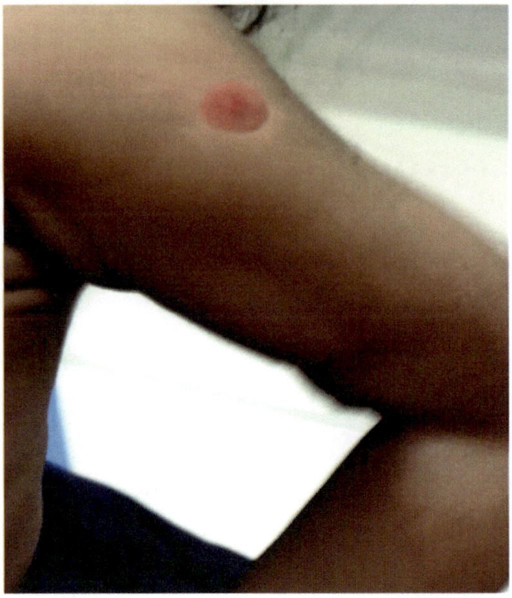

Fig. 11.2 BCG scar reactivation

noted and the BCG scar also showed signs of reactivation (Fig. 11.2). However, there was no other mucosal involvement, rashes, or lymphadenopathy. In view of these findings, irritability and high ESR and CRP, the possibility of Kawasaki disease (KD) was considered.

3. *What is Kawasaki disease and how is the diagnosis made?*

Kawasaki disease is an acute, self-limited medium vessel vasculitis of unknown etiology that occurs in infants and young children. It is a leading cause of acquired heart disease with 25% of untreated patients developing coronary artery aneurysm. Other complications include depressed myocardial contractility and heart failure, myocardial infarction, arrhythmias, and peripheral arterial occlusion, which can result in significant morbidity or even mortality. There is no single pathognomonic clinical feature or diagnostic test. Hence, clinical criteria have been established to help in diagnosing KD. These include:

Fever for 5 days or longer and at least four of the following:

(a) Non-exudative conjunctival injection.

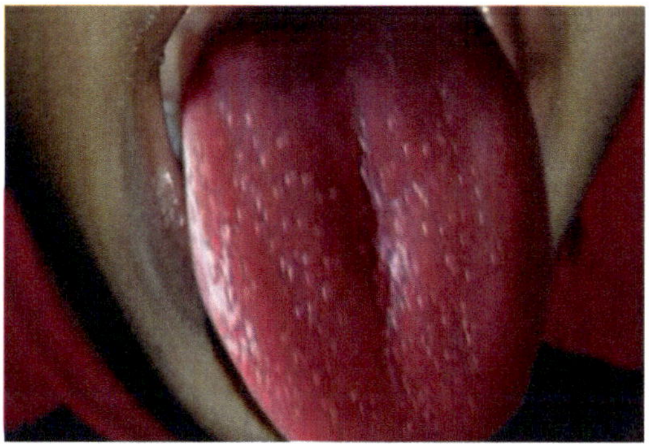

Fig. 11.3 Glossitis (strawberry tongue)

(b) Erythema of oral and pharyngeal mucosa, strawberry tongue (Fig. 11.3), and cracked or erythematous lips.
(c) Erythema/edema of the hands and feet in the acute phase, desquamation during convalescence.
(d) Polymorphous rash.
(e) Unilateral cervical adenopathy >1.5 cm in diameter.

Other findings include arthralgia, dysuria, gastrointestinal symptoms like abdominal pain, vomiting, and diarrhea, inflammation of the BCG vaccination site, and neurological symptoms like irritability.

4. *What is incomplete Kawasaki disease?*

Children often present with clinical features suggestive of KD, without fulfilling all the criteria listed above. The term "incomplete KD" is used in such patients. Incomplete KD is seen more often in infants as they have a lower incidence of lymphadenopathy, rash, and extremity changes, but this is the age group that is at high risk of developing coronary aneurysm. Hence, a high index of suspicion should be maintained. The diagnosis of incomplete KD remains uncertain unless the child develops coronary artery (CA) abnormalities. However, the goal is to identify children at risk who would benefit from treatment for KD before they develop CA abnormalities. Incomplete KD should be suspected, and laboratory evaluation and echocardiography should be performed in patients <6 months of age with unexplained fever ≥7 days, even if there are no clinical findings of KD, and in patients of any age with unexplained fever for ≥5 days, even if only two clinical criteria are present.

5. *What are the investigations useful in making a diagnosis of KD?*

There is no specific diagnostic test, but some laboratory investigations support the diagnosis. Most children have a raised ESR >40 mm/first hour and a raised serum level of CRP >3 mg/dL. The other supportive laboratory criteria are as follows:

(a) Anemia for age.
(b) Platelet count ≥450,000 after the seventh day of fever.
(c) Albumin ≤3.0 g/dL.
(d) Elevated alanine aminotransferase (ALT) level.
(e) WBC count ≥15,000/mm^3.
(f) ≥10 WBC/HPF on urinalysis.

Thrombocytosis is frequently present but only from the second week. Pyuria is a specific feature, occurring in 30–80% of patients with KD, particularly in those ≤1 year of age. In the second week, echocardiographic findings of coronary vasculitis begin to develop.

Blood tests were repeated (day 6 of illness). ESR was 80 mm/h and CRP was 5 mg/dL. Her peripheral leukocyte and thrombocyte counts were 15,200 and 680,000/mL, respectively. Her echocardiography revealed dilatation of both the CAs (2.6 mm left and 3.1 mm right). The +2.5 *Z*-scores of the left and right main coronary artery (CA) were 2.13 and 4.13, respectively. Thus, a diagnosis of incomplete KD was made in the child.

6. *Who are the children at higher risk for developing coronary artery lesions (CAL)?*

The risk factors for coronary artery lesions (CAL) include:

(a) Delayed treatment with intravenous immunoglobulin (IVIG).
(b) Age <1 year and >9 years. Infants, particularly those <6 months, have the highest risk of aneurysms, even with prompt treatment. Also, since many infants present with atypical disease, diagnosis and treatment may be delayed.
(c) Male sex.
(d) Fever for ≥14 days.
(e) Failure to respond to initial IVIG therapy (persistent/recrudescent fever).
(f) Abnormal laboratory findings (low hematocrit (i.e., <35%), low serum albumin (<3 g/dL), low serum sodium (i.e., <135 mEq/L), elevated alanine aminotransferase, elevated white blood cell count (>12,000/mm^3), elevated C-reactive protein, and erythrocyte sedimentation rate).

Identifying children at the highest risk for development of CAL at the time of presentation could guide management decisions but the risk scores developed based on the data from Japanese children have poor sensitivity for predicting IVIG resistance and CAL in other populations.

7. *Does the echocardiography finding of coronary dilatation confirm the diagnosis of KD?*

Mild CA dilatation may be seen in children with other febrile illnesses but a significant dilatation with Z-scores of the left anterior descending coronary artery or right coronary artery being >2.5 is a reliable marker of KD. Echocardiography is also considered positive if three or more of the following features are present: decreased left ventricular function, mitral regurgitation, pericardial effusion, or Z-scores in the left anterior descending coronary artery or right coronary artery of > 2–2.5.

8. *What are the other conditions that can have similar clinical/laboratory features and hence be misdiagnosed as KD before echocardiographic abnormalities develop?*

Fever with rash and similar laboratory abnormalities can be present in some infectious conditions like adenovirus infection and atypical measles as well as noninfectious conditions like sarcoid, polyarteritis nodosa, systemic onset juvenile idiopathic arthritis, drug hypersensitivity, and toxic shock syndrome. Many of these conditions may be misdiagnosed as incomplete KD before the correct diagnosis is made. Also, around one-third of children with KD have a concurrent infection, so even the diagnosis of a concurrent infection does not exclude the diagnosis of KD. During the COVID pandemic, there were many cases of multisystem inflammatory syndrome in children (MIS-C), which was characterized by clinical features similar to those of KD.

9. *Is it likely that incomplete KD may be overdiagnosed and treated?*

Most clinicians would prefer to treat uncertain cases as a safe and effective therapy is available. This is because delay in recognizing and treating incomplete KD would result in the child subsequently developing coronary artery (CA) aneurysms.

10. *How is incomplete KD treated?*

The treatment of incomplete KD is no different from that of KD fulfilling the diagnostic criteria. KD is a self-limited condition, and fever and manifestations of acute inflammation typically resolve in 12 days without therapy. Intravenous immunoglobulin (IVIG) administered within 10 days of fever onset reduces the risk of CA aneurysms from approximately 25% to <5%. It also causes rapid resolution of other signs of inflammation, fever, and lymphocytic myocarditis seen in the disease. The recommended initial therapy includes IVIG (2 g/kg) administered as a single infusion over 8–12 h with aspirin (30–50 mg/kg daily divided into 4 doses) for 5 days or till 48 h after the fever resolves, followed by low-dose aspirin (3–5 mg/kg/day). The duration of low-dose aspirin depends on the extent of coronary artery involvement.

11.2 Conclusion

She was treated with IVIG and aspirin. Her fever and irritability regressed after the IVIG dose. The patient was discharged after 5 days on low-dosage aspirin, 3 mg/kg per day. A gradual regression of the dilatation was observed in the coronary blood vessels on follow-up, and the echocardiographic findings normalized after 2 months.

Learning Points

1. Clinicians caring for children should always consider the possibility of KD when there is unexplained fever lasting for 5 or more days.
2. In infants, incomplete KD is more common than typical KD, and they have a lower incidence of cervical lymphadenopathy, rash, extremity changes, and elevated C-reactive protein.
3. Some infants, especially below 6 months of age, may present only with fever and no other clinical features of KD.
4. The fever in KD is self-limiting, and the diagnosis is sometimes made retrospectively when there is periungual desquamation after resolution of the fever.
5. Children with incomplete KD are more likely to be diagnosed late and are hence at a greater risk of CA aneurysm formation.
6. Early diagnosis and early initiation of IVIG, specifically within 7 days, can decrease the incidence of CA aneurysms from 25% to <5.

Suggested Readings

Idris I, Awadelkarim AM, Saad E, Dayco J, Beker S. Incomplete Kawasaki disease in an infant: a case report and literature review. Cureus. 2022;14(2):e22122. https://doi.org/10.7759/cureus.22122. PMID: 35308689; PMCID: PMC8918302.

McCrindle BW, Rowley AH, Newburger JW, et al. Diagnosis, treatment, and long-term management of Kawasaki disease: a scientific statement for health professionals from the American Heart Association. Circulation. 2017;135:e927.

Singh S, Jindal AK. Kawasaki disease—update. Indian J Pract Pediatr. 2016;18(4):320–7.

Acute Lymphoblastic Leukemia 12

Contents

Key Messages
Pediatricians should maintain a high index of suspicion for acute leukemia in young children with musculoskeletal pain, especially if it awakens the child during sleep. Early in the course of the disease, the total leucocyte count and peripheral smear may be normal.

12.1 Case Discussion

A 3-year-old girl, previously well, presented with a history of fever reaching up to 103 °F for 5 days. The child was responding well to oral paracetamol with fever defervescence. She complained of body aches and preferred to stay in bed. There were no associated chills or rigors. There were no localizing symptoms related to the respiratory, gastrointestinal, or urinary tract. Her appetite had reduced but her urine output was normal. There was no history of fever in her family or among her schoolmates. Past medical or surgical conditions were unremarkable. Her vaccinations were up to date. She was developmentally appropriate for her age.

On physical examination, the child was well grown and conscious but lethargic. Her body temperature was 102.8 °F, respiratory rate was 30 breaths/min, heart rate was 135 beats/min, oxygen saturation was 95% in room air, and blood pressure was 98/73 mmHg. Capillary refill time was 1 s. There were no skin rashes, lymph node enlargement, joint swelling, or deformity. Chest examination revealed equal bilateral air entry, with no added sounds. Cardiovascular examination showed normal first and second heart sounds, no murmur, with no added sounds. The abdomen was soft and nontender with no hepatosplenomegaly. Her neurological examination revealed a well-oriented girl, with no meningeal signs or focal neurological deficits.

P. Venkat Ramanan, R. Padmanabhan, *Fever in Children*,
https://doi.org/10.1007/978-981-97-9967-1_12

1. *What are the clinical possibilities to be considered?*

The differential diagnosis of fever for a short duration has already been discussed in previous chapters.

The initial possibilities considered in this child were dengue fever and enteric fever. She was investigated accordingly. The family was educated about the warning signs, advised to take oral paracetamol, and asked to come back the following day with her investigation reports.

She was brought back after 48 h. Her fever had subsided, but she continued to prefer staying in bed. Her appetite had improved a little and urine output remained normal. On examination, her vital signs were normal. The complete blood count (CBC) done previously on day 5 of fever showed a hemoglobin (Hb) level of 10.5 g/dL, TC 5800 cells/cu mm, DC P23, L 71, and platelet count 84,000/cu mm. Dengue NS1 Ag was negative, but the IgM antibody was positive. Blood and urine cultures were negative.

A diagnosis of dengue fever without warning signs was made. The parents were asked to come back if there were fresh symptoms or if her lethargy did not improve with time. They were advised to give her adequate fluids and monitor her urine output. The child was brought back after 4 days. There was no fever, but she continued to complain of leg pain and sometimes waking up at night crying with pain. On examination, she was afebrile, and her vital signs were normal. She appeared pale and had tenderness over both her legs. There was no joint swelling or restriction of movements. Systemic examination continued to remain normal.

2. *Musculoskeletal pain is a relatively common complaint among children. What is the differential diagnosis and when should such pain be evaluated?*

Though musculoskeletal pains are common in school-aged children, such pain in a child ≤3 years of age should always be investigated. Similarly, pain associated with other clinical findings like fever, pallor, lymphadenopathy, or organomegaly should also be investigated. Other red flag signs in musculoskeletal pains include refusal to walk, night time pain that wakens a child from sleep, pain at rest, swelling/limitation of joint movements, tenderness, and any pain persisting for over 2 weeks.

In dengue fever without complications, children become active once the fever subsides. Given the pallor and significant leg pain, the possibility of a hematological malignancy was considered. Her complete blood count was repeated along with serum LDH levels.

3. *What is the usefulness of serum LDH levels in suspected malignancies?*

Lactate dehydrogenase (LDH) activity is present in all the body cells; when cells die, their LDH is released into the circulating blood. Thus, increased serum LDH level correlates with increased cellular activity, and LDH has been suggested as a tumor marker for many years. Serum LDH levels are increased in almost all malignancies, and higher LDH levels in acute lymphoblastic leukemia (ALL) are associated with high leukocyte counts and blast cells. The total serum LDH level is often increased in malignancies.

Laboratory investigations revealed Hb 9.8 g/dL, TC 7800 cells/cu mm, DC P23, L 71, and platelet count 78,000/cu mm. Peripheral smear examination was also reported to be normal. The serum LDH was 378 U/L (ref. range: upper limit 235 U/L).

4. *How long does thrombocytopenia associated with dengue fever last? Can other infections also cause thrombocytopenia?*

In dengue fever, platelet count usually returns to normal by day 10 of fever. Thrombocytopenia is a recognized complication after infection with other viruses such as Epstein–Barr virus, varicella virus, cytomegalovirus, rubella virus, or hepatitis virus (A, B, or C).

In this child, only the dengue IgM antibody levels were elevated. After an episode of dengue fever, the IgM levels remain elevated typically for 3 months and sometimes even longer. Hence, in this child, the diagnosis of dengue fever is not certain. Because of her persisting thrombocytopenia and elevated serum LDH levels, despite her normal peripheral blood smear, the possibility of a hematological malignancy remained.

5. *Can the total leucocyte count (TLC) and peripheral blood smear be normal in acute leukemia?*

In around half of the children with ALL, the initial CBC may show a TLC of less than 11,000/cmm. So, a normal TLC does not rule out ALL. The peripheral blood smear usually shows blast cells (immature white blood cells) in ALL (Fig. 12.1). But rarely, especially early in the course of the disease when the blast cells multiplying in the marrow are not yet actively released into the bloodstream, the peripheral blood smear may be normal. Hence, if there is a strong clinical suspicion, a bone marrow examination should be done.

Bone marrow aspiration and biopsy were done in the child under sedation. The bone marrow examination revealed numerous blast cells (Fig. 12.2). A diagnosis of acute lymphoblastic leukaemia was made. Flow cytometric analysis was done to confirm the subtype.

6. *What is acute lymphoblastic leukemia?*

Leukemia is a malignancy of the bone marrow and the most common pediatric malignancy. Acute lymphoblastic leukemia (ALL) is responsible for nearly 80% of cases of leukemia in children. The peak incidence is between 3 and 7 years. In acute lymphoblastic leukemia, the lymphoblasts in the bone marrow do not mature, and their unregulated proliferation in the marrow disturbs the production of normal blood cells resulting in cytopenias. Eventually, the lymphoblasts enter the blood and proliferate in the lymph nodes, liver, spleen, and other organs. ALL is classified as B-cell ALL or T-cell ALL, depending on which cell lineage is affected.

7. *Musculoskeletal pains being a feature in both malignancies and rheumatological conditions, are there clinical clues to differentiate between the two conditions?*

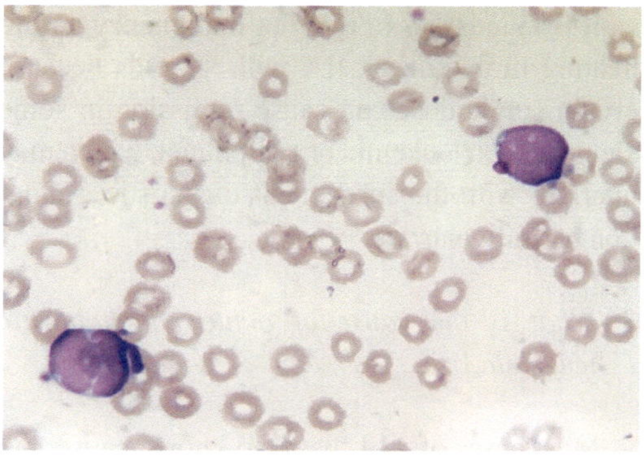

Fig. 12.1 Peripheral blood smear showing blast cells. (Photo Courtesy Dr. S. Sri Gayathri)

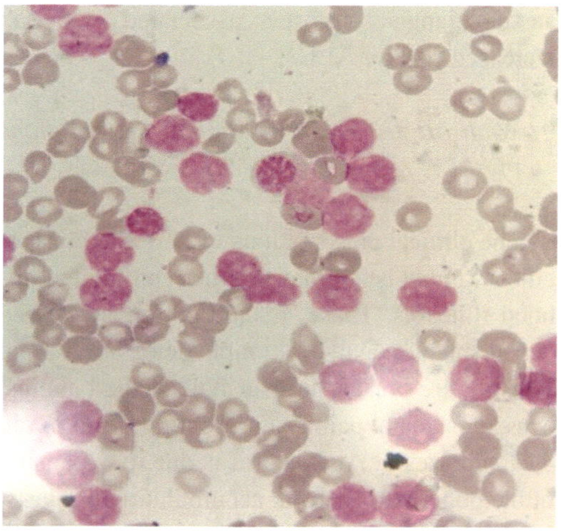

Fig. 12.2 Bone marrow aspirate showing numerous lymphoblasts. (Photo Courtesy Dr. S. Sri Gayathri)

Musculoskeletal pain is a common presenting symptom in approximately 60–70% of children with acute leukemia, but children who are not old enough to verbalize may present with a limp or reluctance to walk. The clinical features help in differentiating between malignancies and rheumatological conditions. Pain in the limbs away from the joints and night pain are more common in leukemia, whereas joint swelling and stiffness, especially in early mornings, occur more commonly in rheumatologic conditions. Laboratory findings such as leukopenia, anemia, thrombocytopenia, and elevated serum lactate dehydrogenase are more common in malignancies. A bone marrow examination should be performed if there is uncertainty about the diagnosis.

It is mandatory to rule out malignancy before treating limb pain as JIA with steroids because even a single dose can cause remission in some children with leukemia or lymphoma, which may interfere with the subsequent diagnostic evaluation of malignancies.

8. *What is the cause of acute lymphoblastic leukemia?*

Most cases of ALL have no known cause, but there are some environmental and genetic risk factors. Genetic syndromes like Down syndrome, neurofibromatosis type 1, Bloom syndrome, and ataxia–telangiectasia are associated with an increased risk for ALL.

9. *What are the common clinical presentations of ALL?*

The clinical presentations of ALL are nonspecific and may be similar to other common childhood illnesses. These include pallor, fever, and hepatosplenomegaly. Lymphadenopathy and bruising are present in over half of the patients. Musculoskeletal pain is a presenting symptom in 43% of cases of ALL, and it is due to expansion of the bone marrow from accumulation of blasts. Young children with bone pain may present with a limp or refusal to bear weight. Leukemia involving the central nervous system can present with headache, vomiting, lethargy, and nuchal rigidity, mimicking meningitis. Painless unilateral testicular enlargement can be a presenting sign of ALL in <1%, but testicular involvement is present in up to 10% of boys with relapsed leukemia. A mediastinal mass, which is most often associated with T-ALL can cause superior vena cava (SVC) syndrome. Respiratory distress can be caused by a mass compressing the trachea.

12.2 Conclusion

The child was referred to the pediatric hemato-oncology unit for further evaluation and management. She was stratified as standard risk after evaluation and treated accordingly. She has tolerated the treatment and responded well to chemotherapy.

Learning Points

1. Pediatricians should maintain a high index of suspicion for acute leukemia in young children with unexplained fever, bone pain, hepatosplenomegaly, and/or lymphadenopathy.
2. ALL should be considered in the differential diagnosis of children with anemia, unexplained lymphocytosis, and cytopenias.
3. Musculoskeletal pain is a common presenting symptom in children with acute leukemia.
4. Early in the course of ALL, the typical findings of lymphadenopathy and organomegaly may not be present.
5. In acute lymphoblastic leukemia (ALL), the peripheral blood smear usually shows blast cells but rarely, it may be normal.
6. Serum LDH levels are often increased in ALL.
7. Children with suspected ALL should be referred promptly to a pediatric hemato-oncology center for diagnosis and management.

Suggested Readings

American Cancer Society. Signs and symptoms of cancer in children. https://www.cancer.org/cancer/cancer-in-children/finding-childhood-cancers-early.html. Accessed 12 Jun 2024.

Civino A, Alighieri G, Prete E, et al. Musculoskeletal manifestations of childhood cancer and differential diagnosis with juvenile idiopathic arthritis (ONCOREUM): a multicentre, cross-sectional study. Lancet Rheumatol. 2021;3:e507.

Clarke RT, Van den Bruel A, Bankhead C, et al. Clinical presentation of childhood leukaemia: a systematic review and meta-analysis. Arch Dis Child. 2016;101:894.

Infectious Mononucleosis 13

Contents

Key Messages
Examination of the throat with a tongue depressor is important when a child presents with fever. When antibiotics are initiated for pharyngitis with exudates and the child does not improve or a maculopapular rash develops, IM should be suspected.

13.1 Case Discussion

A 4-year-old male child presented with fever for 2 days, with the maximum temperature measured being 101 °F. He was otherwise accepting feeds and active. There were no respiratory symptoms or contact with an infected person. His past history included an episode of otitis media which was treated with amoxicillin …months back. Prior to the above presentation, the child was well.

On examination, he was alert and his vital signs were normal. There were no rashes or lymph nodes. Throat examination revealed bilateral hyperemic tonsils (Fig. 13.1).

1. *What are the causes of hyperemic tonsils?*

The most common cause of hyperemic tonsils is tonsillitis, which is commonly due to viruses like rhinovirus, respiratory syncytial virus, adenovirus, coxsackievirus (herpangina), SARS-Cov 2, and Epstein–Barr virus (EBV).

A diagnosis of acute tonsillitis probably viral in etiology was made. He was started on oral paracetamol and asked to be reviewed after 48 h if fever persisted. On review after 48 h, the mother reported that fever persisted, and he was also not taking oral feeds well. On examination, the sensorium was normal, and vitals were maintained. Child had bilaterally palpable, mildly tender, and firm posterior cervical lymph nodes (Fig. 13.2). Eye and ear examination and neck movements were normal. Throat examination revealed bilaterally enlarged tonsils with exudates (Fig. 13.3). There were no palatal petechiae or ulcers in the oral cavity.

Exudative tonsillitis could be caused by viral (adenovirus, EBV) or bacterial pathogens (Group A *Streptococcus*, diphtheria). Streptococcal pharyngitis is the most common

P. Venkat Ramanan, R. Padmanabhan, *Fever in Children*,
https://doi.org/10.1007/978-981-97-9967-1_13

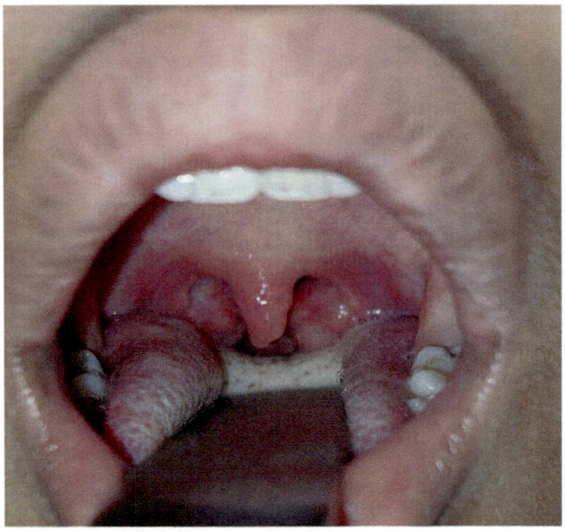

Fig. 13.1 Bilateral enlarged hyperemic tonsils. (Photo Courtesy Dr. S. Prasanna Kumar)

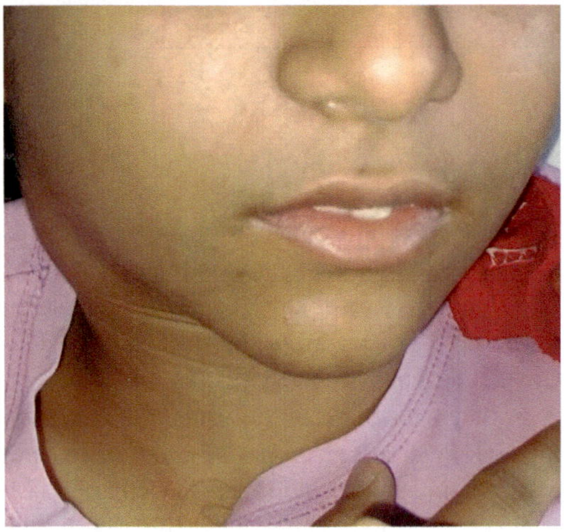

Fig. 13.2 Posterior cervical lymphadenopathy. (Photo Courtesy Dr. S. Prasanna Kumar)

bacterial cause. In diphtheria, a thick adherent membrane (like exudate) which bleeds on separation is seen, with significant enlargement of the cervical lymph nodes ("bull neck"). In infectious mononucleosis (IM), large, mildly tender posterior cervical lymph nodes, diffuse lymphadenopathy outside the cervical region, and splenomegaly or, less commonly, hepatomegaly may be seen.

A diagnosis of acute tonsillitis probably due to Group A beta hemolytic *Streptococcus* (GABHS) was made in view of tonsillar enlargement with exudates and the absence of cough and other

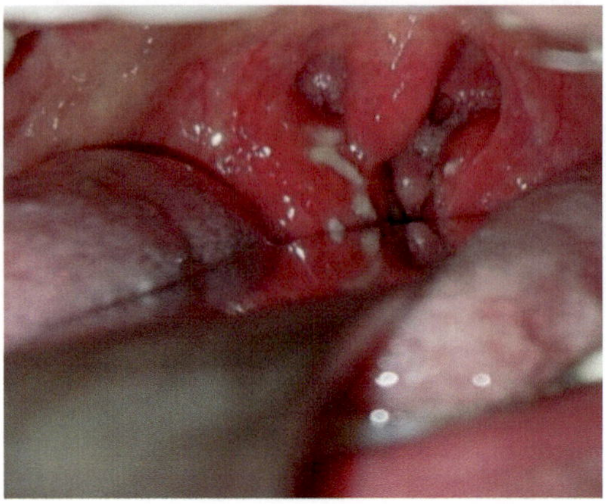

Fig. 13.3 Exudative tonsillitis. (Photo Courtesy Dr. S. Prasanna Kumar)

mucosal involvement. A throat swab was sent for culture, and the child was started on amoxicillin and asked to review after 48 h.

2. *When should GABHS be suspected as the cause of tonsillitis?*

Most episodes of tonsillitis are caused by viruses. Group A beta-hemolytic streptococcus (GABHS), the most common bacterial etiology, accounts for 15–30% of acute tonsillitis in children, usually in the age group of 5–15 years. Cough, coryza, and diarrhea are more common with viral pharyngitis, while sore throat without cough, sudden onset of fever greater than 100.4 °F [38 °C], anterior cervical lymphadenopathy, and tonsillar inflammation or exudates are common in GABHS. Clinical findings alone cannot be relied upon, and diagnostic tests are recommended (throat culture/rapid antigen detection tests).

The parents came back after 48 h with persistent fever. Throat culture was sterile. He had developed pain on swallowing, drooling of saliva, and a maculopapular rash on face and trunk (Fig. 13.4). A systemic examination was done which showed hepatomegaly (liver palpable 3 cm below costal margin). There was no splenomegaly, and the rest of the systems were normal.

3. *What is the differential diagnosis that should be considered now?*

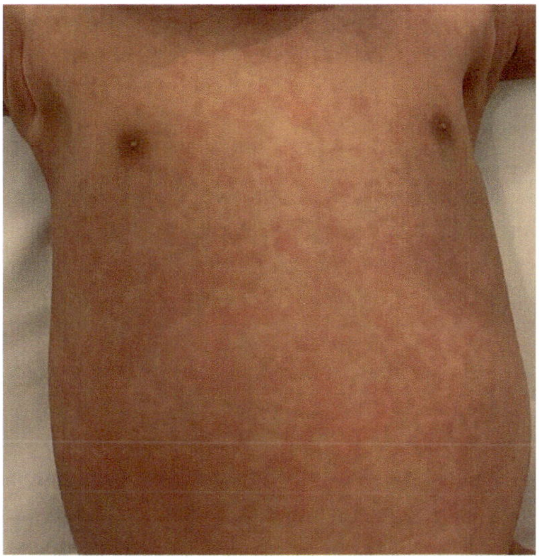

Fig. 13.4 Maculopapular rash over trunk after starting amoxicillin. (Photo courtesy Dr. Dhanaratnamoorthy)

In pharyngitis caused by GABHS, the symptoms are expected to improve once treatment with appropriate antibiotics is initiated. Amoxicillin is known to cause drug rash, but this child had been previously treated with amoxicillin without any allergies. Historically, ampicillin and amoxicillin administration have been reported to precipitate a maculopapular rash in most adolescents with IM but is less common in children. Recent studies indicate that rash is seen with the same frequency in those patients with IM who did not receive any drug and is believed to be due to virus-mediated vasculitis.

A provisional diagnosis of infectious mononucleosis (IM) was made, and the child was hospitalized. Intravenous fluids and analgesics were started, and antibiotics were stopped.

4. *What is Infectious mononucleosis (IM)?*

IM is a clinical syndrome caused by Epstein–Barr virus (EBV) infection. Young children acquire the virus from asymptomatic parents or siblings through contact with oropharyngeal secretions, and the infection is usually subclinical during childhood years. In developing countries, EBV seroprevalence is almost 100% by 4 years of age. In developed countries, the infection is usually acquired during adolescence or early adulthood. The infection persists lifelong, and reactivation is possible whenever the immune system weakens.

5. *What are the clinical features to suspect IM?*

Fever, sore throat, lymphadenopathy, and tonsillopharyngitis are the classic clinical features of IM. Rash is usually maculopapular and is seen more commonly in preschool children (34%) than in children older than 4 years (17%).

6. *What investigations can help diagnose IM?*
   (a) A complete blood count (CBC) is indicated and the following reports suggest a diagnosis of IM:
      - A white blood cell (WBC) count of 12,000–18,000 cells/mm^3 with lymphocytosis (absolute count >4500 cells/mm^3 or a differential count >50%). At times, mild neutropenia and thrombocytopenia may be present, which is self-limiting. Rarely, patients may develop hemolytic anemia and hemophagocytic lymphohistiocytosis.
      - Peripheral smear showing significant atypical lymphocytosis (>10% of total lymphocytes). Atypical lymphocytes are larger lymphocytes with irregular nuclear shapes and abundant cytoplasm. Basophilic stippling or vacuolation also may be seen. These are seen in viral infections (EBV, cytomegalovirus, hepatitis virus), bacterial infections (pertussis, tuberculosis, toxoplasmosis), autoimmune disorders (systemic lupus erythematosus, rheumatoid arthritis), and intake of certain drugs (phenytoin, carbamazepine).
      - Raised aminotransferases in a child with pharyngitis should always alert the clinician to a strong diagnostic possibility of IM.

   (b) The diagnosis must be confirmed by heterophile antibody test (monospot) or by

EBV-specific antibodies. Monospot test is a latex agglutination assay, and if positive, further confirmation is not necessary. It is, however, often negative in children less than 4 years; hence, EBV-specific antibodies (IgG and IgM) to viral capsid antigen (VCA) must be tested in this age group. These antibodies are present on day 1 of clinical illness due to the long incubation period (2–4 weeks). IgM levels decrease 3 months later, while IgG persists for life. IgG antibodies to EBV nuclear antigen (EBNA) appear 6–12 weeks after the onset of symptoms and persist throughout life. Their presence early in an illness rules out acute EBV infection. Hence, a positive VCA antibody test with negative EBNA antibody test is diagnostic of IM.

Investigations were sent and reports are as follows: CBC showed a total leukocyte count of 21,340 cells/cmm^3. There were 62% lymphocytes, 37% neutrophils, and 1% eosinophils. The absolute lymphocyte count was 13,230 cells/cmm^3. Hemoglobin and platelet counts were normal. C-reactive protein level was less than 5 mg/L. Peripheral smear examination revealed atypical lymphocytes (Fig. 13.5), which constituted 11% of total cells. No abnormal cells were seen. Liver function test was normal. EBV-specific antibodies to VCA (IgG and IgM) were sent.

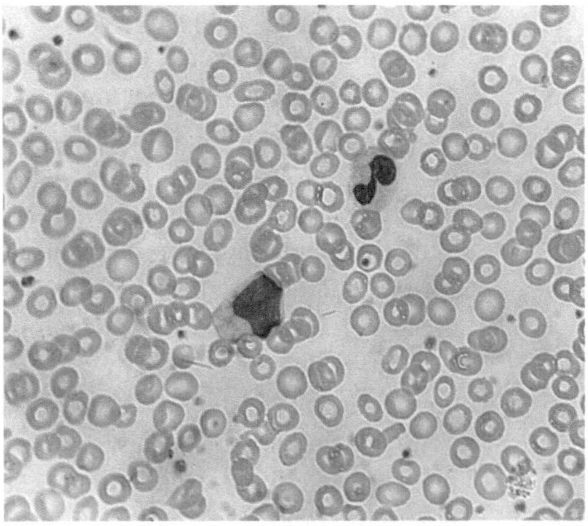

Fig. 13.5 Peripheral smear showing atypical lymphocytes. (Photo courtesy Dr. Srigayathri)

7. *How is IM treated?*

Management is supportive with antipyretics and adequate hydration. Antibiotics and antivirals have no role. In children with impending airway obstruction, corticosteroids may be used.

8. *What is the usefulness of establishing a lab diagnosis if there is no specific treatment?*

Diagnosis is useful as serious complications like splenic rupture and airway obstruction can be anticipated and informed to caregivers. Besides, with a specific diagnosis of EBV infection, unnecessary antibiotic therapy is avoided.

13.2 Conclusion

EBV VCA IgM titers were >160 U/mL (reference range <40), and IgG was 40 U/mL (reference range <20). The throat swab and blood culture were sterile after 48 h. A final diagnosis of IM was

Learning Points

1. Fever, sore throat, posterior cervical lymphadenopathy, and tonsillopharyngitis are the classic clinical features of IM.
2. Tonsillitis in young children is most commonly viral but bacterial tonsillitis by GABHS should be ruled out.
3. A maculopapular rash is seen more commonly in preschool children (34%) with IM than in children older than 4 years (17%).
4. Historically, amoxicillin administration has been reported to precipitate the rash, and it is believed to be a transient virus-mediated immune alteration, resulting in the development of a reversible, delayed-type hypersensitivity reaction to the antibiotic.

5. Recent studies indicate that rash is seen with the same frequency in those patients with IM who did not receive any drug and is believed to be due to virus-mediated vasculitis.
6. Typically, a white blood cell (WBC) count of 12,000–18,000 cells/mm^3 with lymphocytosis and a peripheral smear showing significant atypical lymphocytosis (>10% of total lymphocytes) are seen.
7. The diagnosis is confirmed by serology. EBV-specific antibodies (IgG and IgM) to viral capsid antigen (VCA) are present on day 1 of clinical illness due to the long incubation period (2–4 weeks). IgM levels decrease 3 months later, while IgG persists throughout life.

made, and the child was managed with supportive care. As his activity and oral intake improved, he was discharged after 3 days of hospital stay.

Suggested Readings

Ali AS, Al-Shraim M, Al-Hakami AM, Jones IM. Epstein-Barr Virus: clinical and epidemiological revisits and genetic basis of oncogenesis. Open Virol J. 2015;9:7–28.

Ebell MH. Epstein-Barr virus infectious mononucleosis. Am Fam Physician. 2004;70(7):1279–86.

Luzuriaga K, Sullivan JL. Infectious mononucleosis. N Engl J Med. 2010;362:1993.

Drug Fever

14

Contents

> **Key Messages**
> Drug fever (DF) is not uncommon and should be considered in the differential diagnosis of nosocomial fever and fever of unknown origin. Failure to recognize DF by clinicians may result in prolonged hospitalization, unnecessary investigation, and medications.

14.1 Case Discussion

A 2-year-old girl presented with high-grade fever for 4 days and abdominal pain with vomiting for 2 days. There was no history of respiratory or genitourinary symptoms. She had no known drug allergies. There was a history of urinary tract infection (UTI) twice in the past which was treated with intravenous (IV) ceftriaxone followed by oral cefixime. Her micturating cystourethrogram and dimercaptosuccinic acid (DMSA) scans were normal. On physical examination, she was uncomfortable and ill-appearing. Her body temperature was 101.2 °F, pulse rate was 98 bpm, and blood pressure was 92/70 mmHg. On examination of the abdomen, there was right lumbar tenderness. All other systems were normal on examination. The initial laboratory reports revealed a hemoglobin level of 11.4 g/dL, total leucocyte cell count (TLC) of 18,900/cmm with 74% neutrophils, platelet count of 2.3 lacs/cmm, erythrocyte sedimentation rate (ESR) of 34 mm/h, and C-reactive protein (CRP) level of 65 mg/L. The child's electrolytes were within the normal range, and renal and liver function tests were normal. Urine routine examination revealed 18 pus cells per high power field. A diagnosis of upper urinary tract infection was made. A catheter urine sample was sent for culture

1. *How can lower tract infection be differentiated from upper tract infection?*

Lower tract infection (cystitis) is characterized by voiding-related symptoms like burning micturition, increased frequency of voiding, and urgency. Fever and other systemic signs may or may not be present. Upper tract infection

P. Venkat Ramanan, R. Padmanabhan, *Fever in Children*,
https://doi.org/10.1007/978-981-97-9967-1_14

(pyelonephritis) presents with fever, flank pain, chills, nausea, vomiting, and anorexia, and voiding-related symptoms may be absent especially in children <2 years. In young children, it is difficult to differentiate pyelonephritis from cystitis. Febrile UTI should be assumed to be pyelonephritis and treated accordingly. In febrile UTI, an erythrocyte sedimentation rate (ESR) of more than 30 mm/h and elevated C-reactive protein (CRP) levels are sensitive, but nonspecific markers of renal parenchymal involvement. An ultrasound of the kidneys, ureters, and bladder (USG KUB) is useful for determining the size and shape of the kidneys and to exclude congenital malformations in children; but, it has low sensitivity (50%) in detecting acute pyelonephritis. Focal abnormalities on ultrasonography with elevated CRP level may be predictive of renal scarring.

An abdominal USG revealed enlarged kidneys with a hypoechoic parenchyma and loss of the normal corticomedullary differentiation.

2. *What is the recommended treatment for acute pyelonephritis?*

Upper urinary tract infection is treated initially with parenteral antibiotics. Most cases of acute pyelonephritis in children are caused by *Escherichia coli* or *Klebsiella pneumoniae*, and over 80% of these organisms in South India produce extended-spectrum beta-lactamase (ESBL). Because of high resistance rates to cephalosporins reported, the initial treatment should include a beta-lactam–beta-lactamase inhibitor combination (BL-BLI), trimethoprim–sulfamethoxazole (TMP-SMZ), or aminoglycoside. Therapy is initiated with IV antibiotics till the child becomes asymptomatic and is followed by oral therapy to complete a 10–14-day course.

The child was started on IV piperacillin–tazobactam. Over the next 72 h, the abdominal pain and vomiting subsided, the fever became low grade, and the child became playful. Her urine grew extended spectrum beta lactamase (ESBL) producing *Klebsiella*. The urine culture report is shown in Fig. 14.1.

IV piperacillin–tazobactam was continued with a plan to switch over to oral antibiotics once the child was asymptomatic. On day 6 of antibiotics, high-grade fever spikes restarted with a maximum temperature of 102.2 °F.

3. *What are the causes of fever recurrence in a child who was initially responding to antibiotics?*

Fever recurrence could be due to reinfection with another organism. Sometimes complicating factors like a kidney stone or anatomical abnor-

Fig. 14.1 Urine culture report showing ESBL producing *Klebsiella*

CULTURE & SENSITIVITY - URINE

COLONY COUNT	>10^5 cfu/ml	
Organism I	**Klebsiella pneumoniae (ESBL)**	
Antibiotics	**Disc diffusion**	**MIC(mcg/ml)**
Amoxy/clav	Resistant	
Ciprofloxacin	Intermediate	
Nitrofurantoin	Sensitive	
Gentamycin	Sensitive	
Amikacin	Sensitive	
Cotrimoxazole	Sensitive	
Cefuroxime	Resistant	
Cefixime	Resistant	
Ceftazidime	Resistant	
Piperacillin/tazo	Sensitive	
Cefaperazone/sul	Sensitive	
COMMENT	High resistance pattern noted	

malities make eradication of the organism difficult though in such cases fever is unlikely to subside initially. It could also be because of thrombophlebitis or a secondary infection.

On re-examination, there was no thrombophlebitis or any other focus of infection. The child was re-investigated. CBC showed a TLC of 8460 cells/cmm with 54% neutrophils. Repeat USG KUB did not show any complications. Urinalysis and serum procalcitonin levels were normal. Repeat blood and urine cultures were sterile. Intermittent fever persisted, but she continued to remain playful and active and improve clinically. There was no rash or eosinophilia. It was observed that her pulse rate was between 82 and 94 bpm even during fever spikes. The possibility of drug fever (DF) was considered.

4. *What is drug fever and what are the risk factors for developing drug fever?*

Drug fever (DF) is fever that begins after administration of a drug and resolves within 72 h of discontinuation of the drug without any other therapy, with no other identifiable cause for the fever and no relapse 72 h after defervescence. DF is responsible for 3–7% of all PUO. Fever may be associated with other adverse drug reactions (ADRs) such as skin manifestations, hepatitis, interstitial nephritis, and acute lung injury. A genetic predisposition to drug fever has been described for certain drugs (carbamazepine, allopurinol). Certain viral infections can increase the risk of drug hypersensitivities, especially HIV infection. Infections with cytomegalovirus, Epstein–Barr virus, and human herpes virus 6 are also associated with an increased risk of drug hypersensitivity. Patients with cystic fibrosis are reported to have a high incidence of antibiotic-associated drug fever, in particular with piperacillin and imipenem–cilastatin.

5. *What is the lag time between initiation of the culprit drug and the fever onset?*

DF may develop immediately following initiation of therapy but more commonly is delayed for 5–7 days. The time interval can vary widely depending on the type of drug. For antibiotics, the time interval is 1–2 weeks and for antineoplastic agents it is 3–4 days. The time interval is shortened if the patient has received the same class of drugs previously.

6. *What is the mechanism by which drugs cause fever?*

The most common mechanism is drug hypersensitivity. An immune response is triggered with the drug acting as an antigen. In a Jarisch–Herxheimer reaction, the bacteria destroyed by the antibiotic (penicillin) release endotoxins causing an abrupt onset of fever with myalgia 6–8 h after starting the antibiotic. It is associated with increased levels of interleukin-1 (IL-1), IL-6, and tumor necrosis factor. Classically, this reaction was described following the treatment for secondary and tertiary syphilis, brucellosis, and enteric fever.

Drugs can also induce fever by an extension of their pharmacological action such as by increasing heat production (salicylate intoxication and thyroxine), by reducing sweating (e.g., anticholinergic drugs), or by inducing vasoconstriction (adrenaline). Chemotherapeutic drugs cause cell lysis and pyrogenic substances are released from damaged cells; the resulting inflammatory response with cytokine activation causes fever. Fever typically starts 3–4 days after chemotherapy and may last for a week or longer. Cytotoxic drugs also cause immunosuppression with subsequent infections causing febrile episodes, but this develops after the second week of chemotherapy.

Malignant hyperthermia is a rare condition in which there is sudden appearance of fever over 40 °C, muscle rigidity, and hypotension during general anesthesia triggered by muscle relaxants (succinylcholine) and inhaled anesthetic agents (halothane). It usually occurs with the third exposure but can occur with the first exposure also. It is more common in children below 15 years of age and is inherited as an autosomal dominant trait in 50% of cases. Neuroleptic malignant syndrome (high fever, muscle rigidity, altered mental state, and dysautonomia) is caused by CNS dopamine-depleting drugs such as haloperidol that alter hypothalamic thermoregulation.

Fever can also accompany a chemical phlebitis caused by drug administration (e.g., as with cephalothin or potassium chloride), and local inflammation and/or sterile abscesses can occur at sites of injection.

7. *Which drugs can cause drug fever?*

Almost any drug may cause DF, but some drugs are more commonly implicated. These include antibiotics, anticonvulsants, antiarrhythmics (quinidine and procainamide), and cytotoxic drugs. Antimicrobials (beta-lactams, sulfonamides, and nitrofurantoin) are the most common cause of drug fever, responsible for approximately one-third of the episodes. With anticonvulsants (carbamazepine, phenytoin, and phenobarbital), fever may be accompanied by lymphadenopathy and may even cause a lymphoma-like syndrome. When the drug is discontinued, fever and lymphadenopathy resolve slowly in 2–6 weeks. Anticonvulsants may also be associated with eosinophilia and systemic symptoms (drug rash with eosinophilia and systemic symptoms—DRESS syndrome).

8. *What are the clinical clues to the presence of drug fever?*

Bradycardia is the most common symptom of drug fever. In most conditions causing fever, the pulse rate increases by 10 beats per minute for every 1 °F (approximately 0.55 °C) increase in body temperature. This correlation between fever and pulse rate has not been observed in most cases of drug fever, and the absence of relative bradycardia may help rule out drug fever. Another clue is that the general condition of the child is good despite the fever. The fever may be associated with maculopapular or urticaria skin rashes in 15–30%. Patients with maculopapular rashes typically exhibit symmetrical rashes on the entire body. Though chills and rigors are strongly associated with bacteremia, they can also occur in drug fever. Headache and arthralgia may also occur in drug fever. The fever pattern and severity of temperature rise in cases of drug fever are variable. Continuous but fluctuating fever characterized by wide swings that do not return to baseline temperature is the most common fever pattern, but intermittent and remittent fevers can also occur. Fever intensity varies from low grade to high grade and generally has no bearing on prognosis. Muscle rigidity, dysautonomia, agitation, and confusion are clues to the presence of an idiosyncratic reaction, such as neuroleptic malignant syndrome or serotonin syndrome. Drug fever occurs more frequently in certain patient populations, such as people with HIV or cystic fibrosis. Drug fever due to an antimicrobial agent can cause clinical confusion; recurrence of fever in a patient who has defervesced on antimicrobial treatment for an infection may be misinterpreted as relapse of the original infection.

9. *What investigations can help in the diagnosis?*

Drug fever is generally a diagnosis of exclusion. Depending on the clinical situation, investigations to rule out all other causes of fever, such as infection, malignancy, autoimmune or autoinflammatory conditions, and endocrine disorders may be needed. Though there are no diagnostic tests for drug fever, leukocytosis with eosinophilia (in around 25%) may be present. If pyuria is present on urine microscopy, a stain for eosinophils should be performed. Eosinophiluria suggests interstitial nephritis, which is associated with drug fever. Serum procalcitonin, a useful marker of bacteremia, remains low in drug fever. Other laboratory findings include elevated liver enzyme levels, renal failure, or anemia. Inflammatory markers, like C-reactive protein (CRP) and erythrocyte sedimentation rate (ESR), can be normal or increased in drug fever.

10. *When should drug fever be suspected as the cause of fever?*

There is no single clinical feature that can diagnose or exclude drug fever. Drug fever should be considered in the differential diagnosis of new-onset fever, after an afebrile period of more than 48 h during any drug treatment. It should also be considered when there is prolonged fever, for more than 72 h despite appropriate treatment for febrile illnesses. Evaluation of patients with suspected drug fever should include a thorough history and physical examination to identify the cause of the fever. A single administration of a drug can also induce drug fever, and hence a history of drugs that are "used-as-needed" should be obtained. All the current medications, doses, and durations of use should be noted. A past history of drug fever, especially with a medication related to the one the patient is currently taking, should increase the suspicion for drug fever. While most cases occur within the first few weeks of drug initiation, clinicians should be aware that even medications that the patient has been using chronically can be potential causes of DF.

11. *What is the treatment for DF?*

Once a tentative diagnosis of drug fever is made, the drug that is considered to be the cause should be stopped. Drug discontinuation is both diagnostic and therapeutic. If the diagnosis is correct, the fever will usually alleviate within 72 h, the diagnosis is confirmed, and no specific treatment is necessary. If fever continues for longer than 72 h after discontinuation of the drug, the patient should be evaluated for organ-specific symptoms such as liver injury, renal failure, and rashes. Severe organ involvement is treated with corticosteroids. When the patient is on several drugs, the drugs should be stopped individually every 2–3 days, beginning with the most likely drug. If the fever doesn't resolve, sequential cessation of other drugs will be needed. The first drug can be restarted, if necessary. Discontinuing all medications at once may eliminate the fever but the causative drug cannot be identified. Also, the patient may be at some risk from the underlying disease.

12. *When is rechallenge to confirm or rule out a suspected drug needed?*

If discontinuation of the suspected drug does not affect the patient's outcome, rechallenge is not advisable as it involves some risks. If the drugs concerned are the key drugs of treatment (e.g., antitubercular drugs), rechallenge to identify the causative drug may have to be considered. Rechallenge should only be performed when the original drug reaction was not associated with organ damage, blistering skin reactions, or mucous membrane involvement. Drug rechallenge may be harmful and should be performed with extreme caution in a controlled environment where the patient can be closely monitored. The duration of monitoring depends on the initial reaction and how long after initial dosing the fever occurred. The recurrence of fever (usually within a day) with drug rechallenge helps in establishing the diagnosis and causality.

14.2 Conclusion

Piperacillin/tazobactam was discontinued. The temperature normalized within 48 h with no relapse of fever 72 h after defervescence. The antibiotic course was completed with oral trimethoprim-sulfamethoxazole (TMP-SMZ).

Learning Points

1. Drug fever should be considered in the differential diagnosis of nosocomial fever and fever of unknown origin.
2. The typical presentation of DF is recurrence of fever after initial defervescence in a child taking an antibiotic for an infection that is resolving.
3. There is no characteristic fever pattern; it may be a continuous intermittent or remittent fever.
4. The patients usually do not appear toxic, and the body temperature ranges from 38.8 °C (102 °F) to 40.0 °C (104 °F).
5. The drugs most commonly associated with DF are antibacterials (particularly β-lactam antibiotics, sulfa) and antiepileptics.

6. Relative bradycardia is one of the most important diagnostic clues.
7. The lag time between the initiation of the offending agent and the onset of fever is highly variable.
8. The fever may be associated with maculopapular or urticarial skin rashes in 18–29%.
9. The eosinophil count and hepatic transaminases are sometimes raised.
10. Rechallenge is generally discouraged.

The child was referred to the nephrologist for evaluation of recurrent UTI.

Suggested Readings

Patel RA, Gallagher JC. Drug fever. Pharmacotherapy. 2010;30:57.

Someko H, Kataoka Y, Obara T. Drug fever: a narrative review. Ann Clin Epidemiol. 2023;5(4):95–106. https://doi.org/10.37737/ace.23013. PMID: 38504950; PMCID: PMC10944987.

Systemic Juvenile Idiopathic Arthritis

15

Contents

Key Messages
In a young child with PUO, with the typical quotidian fever pattern, SJIA should be considered even in the absence of arthritis. Elevated serum ferritin, inflammatory markers, and FDG-PET/CT scan may play a useful role in making the diagnosis.

15.1 Case Discussion

A 5-year-old boy was referred to our hospital with a history of high-grade, intermittent fever for 7 days, without any localizing symptoms. He had been treated with a course of amoxicillin for 5 days with no response. His past medical history was uneventful. He was fully immunized according to the IAP immunization schedule including the typhoid conjugate vaccine. General physical examination showed the child to be well-appearing with no abnormalities, and systemic examination was normal.

A diagnosis of probable enteric fever or viral infection was made, and blood tests including a complete blood count, cultures, and serological testing for dengue, scrub typhus, and leptospirosis were sent. Since he was otherwise well-appearing, he was started on paracetamol and asked to review on the following day with the reports.

On review, fever was persisting. Blood tests revealed a normal hemoglobin level and peripheral smear, a total leucocyte count (TLC) of 17,600/cu mm with 72% polymorphs, a platelet count of 386,000/cu mm, ESR of 67 mm/first hour, and CRP of 32 mg/dL.

1. *What is the differential diagnosis of a high-grade fever for 8 days with laboratory reports as described above?*

In view of the intermittent nature of fever and polymorphonuclear leukocytosis, the possibility of enteric fever becomes less likely. The high normal platelet count and a relatively well-appearing child on day 8 of fever make dengue and scrub typhus also unlikely. The differentials would be occult infections and noninfectious

P. Venkat Ramanan, R. Padmanabhan, *Fever in Children*,
https://doi.org/10.1007/978-981-97-9967-1_15

conditions like autoimmune disease and malignancy.

A diagnosis of probable occult bacterial infection was made. The child was hospitalized for parenteral antibiotics and for further evaluation. Serological testing results for dengue, scrub typhus, and leptospirosis were negative. Chest X-ray and abdominal ultrasound were normal. Blood and urine cultures were sterile. The high-grade intermittent fever continued with a maximum temperature of 106 °F (Fig. 15.1). On day 3 of hospitalization (day 11 of fever), he started complaining of malaise and generalized body pain, more in the knees during the episodes of fever. There were no new findings on clinical examination, and musculoskeletal examination revealed no signs of arthritis. In between the fever episodes, he was well-appearing and had no pain.

2. *What are the causes of body/joint pain with fever in children?*

Joint pain and body pain in children with fever are nonspecific symptoms and can be present in a wide range of infectious and noninfectious conditions. These include bacterial bone and joint infections, viral or post-infectious arthralgia, rheumatic fever, connective tissue disorders, and malignancy.

Bacterial bone and joint infections may present with high-grade fever, bone/joint pain and swelling, leukocytosis, and elevated inflammatory markers. But the fever is likely to be persistent, and there will be severe localized tenderness over the affected bone or joint. Generally, it is a monoarthritis.

Viral infections like chikungunya and parvovirus B19 can cause fever and a transient arthritis. Post-infectious reactive arthritis may also follow a variety of infections. Rheumatic fever and subacute bacterial endocarditis also present with fever and arthritis. The fever is usually low grade and cardiac involvement may coexist.

Arthralgia/arthritis with fever may be the initial presentation of inflammatory bowel disease (IBD), Kawasaki disease (KD), and several autoimmune and auto-inflammatory diseases.

Fever, bone pain, and joint swelling are also seen in leukemia, and the pain may be fleeting, shifting from one site to another. Refusal to bear weight because of pain and severe pain disturbing night sleep are indicative of a malignancy. The associated thrombocytopenia, lymphocytosis, or neutropenia may give a clue.

Early morning joint stiffness and easing of pain as the day goes on are characteristic of juvenile idiopathic arthritis. Repeated clinical examination and appropriate investigations are needed to reach a diagnosis as the disease evolves and becomes identifiable.

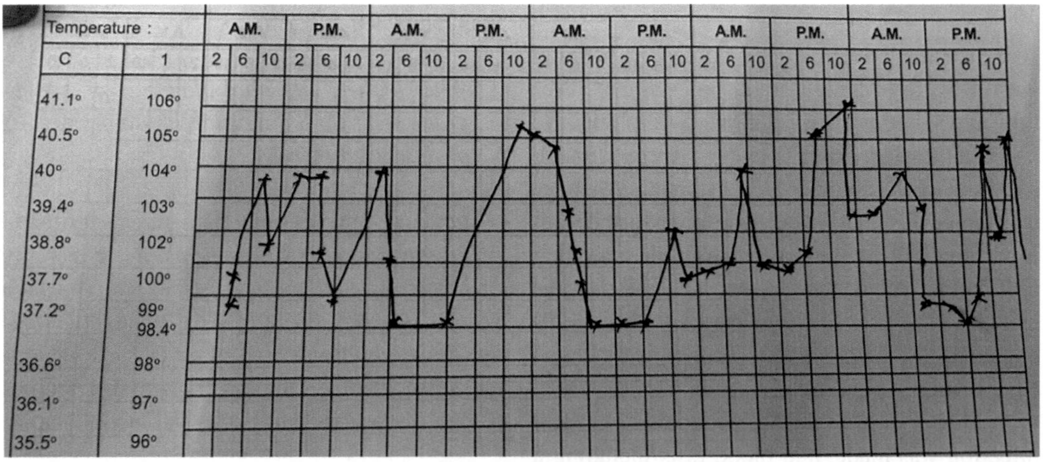

Fig. 15.1 Temperature chart showing quotidian fever (daily fever spikes returning to normal). (Photo courtesy Dr. P. Ramachandran)

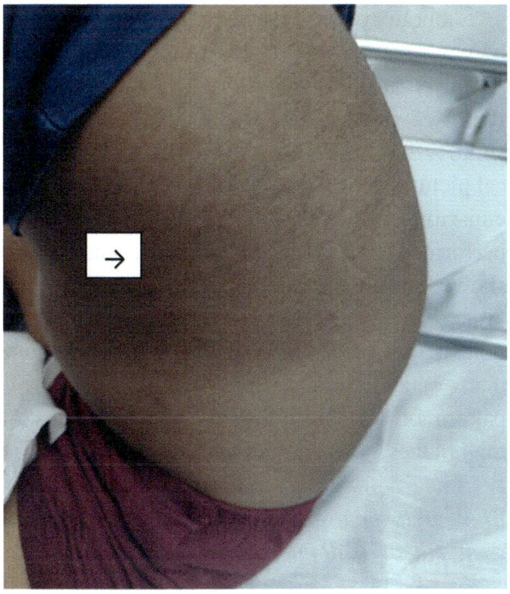

Fig. 15.2 Faint maculopapular rash on the trunk. (Photo courtesy Dr. Mahesh Janardhanan)

Repeat blood tests showed that the inflammatory markers had further increased. The total leukocyte count (TLC) was 24,700/cu mm with 76% polymorphs, erythrocyte sedimentation rate (ESR) was 78 mm/first hour, and C-reaction protein (CRP) was 44 mg/dL. Extensive evaluation for various infectious diseases was negative. Bone marrow aspiration, biopsy, echocardiogram, and CT scans of thorax and abdomen did not reveal any abnormality.

On day 13 of fever, during one of the fever spikes a faint, reddish maculopapular rash was noted over his trunk (Fig. 15.2). The rash disappeared with fever defervescence and reappeared with subsequent fever spikes.

In view of the fever pattern, rashes, joint pain, neutrophilic leukocytosis, raised CRP and ESR, and other investigations being normal, the possibility of systemic juvenile idiopathic arthritis (SJIA) was considered, though the fever duration was only 13 days and the diagnostic criteria were not met.

3. *When should SJIA be considered in the differential diagnosis of PUO?*

SJIA should be suspected when there is high-grade, intermittent fever (≥101.3 °F) for over 2 weeks with malaise, serositis, and joint pain. The joints typically affected are the wrists, knees, and ankles, but the fingers, hips, cervical spine, and temporomandibular joints may also be involved. Typically, there is one fever spike per day that subsides spontaneously and the child remains afebrile during the rest of the 24-h period (quotidian fever). The pain and malaise are present only during the fever spikes. A maculopapular rash tends to appear or worsen during the fever spike. The rash often fades as the temperature returns to normal and reappears with the next spike. Hepatomegaly, splenomegaly, and lymphadenopathy may also be present.

The International League of Associations for Rheumatology (ILAR), has defined SJIA as a disease starting before the age of 16 years, with at least 15 days of fever, a peculiar spiking fever pattern, arthritis persisting for 6 weeks, and at least two of the following features: skin rash, serositis (pericarditis in most cases), lymphadenopathy, hepatomegaly, or splenomegaly. This is because many other conditions (described above) can cause fever and joint pains which resolve in less than 6 weeks. Recently, less stringent criteria to allow earlier diagnosis have been proposed but they are yet to be validated.

SJIA may be difficult to diagnose because the arthritis and rash may not be evident early in the course of the disease, the fever pattern may not be typical, and there are no specific diagnostic tests. Often, it is a diagnosis of exclusion that is considered after infections and malignancy have been ruled out. Any patient suspected of having SJIA should be referred early to pediatric rheumatologists, who are often able to make a diagnosis and begin appropriate therapy before 6 weeks of arthritis have elapsed.

4. *What investigations can help in making a diagnosis of SJIA?*

There are no tests that are specific for the diagnosis, but the laboratory abnormalities that may point to the diagnosis are as follows:

(a) Raised erythrocyte sedimentation rate (ESR) which may exceed 100 mm/h.
(b) Elevated levels of C-reactive protein (CRP).
(c) Anemia due to decreased synthesis, poor absorption of oral iron, and gastrointestinal blood loss induced by nonsteroidal anti-inflammatory drugs (NSAIDs) causing iron deficiency.
(d) Leukocytosis with polymorphonuclear predominance. The total leucocyte count in typically 20,000–30,000/cmm, and sometimes a leukemoid reaction with counts going up to 60,000–80,000/c mm may be seen.
(e) Thrombocytosis, with a platelet count of 500,000–800,000/cmm. Hence, if the platelet count is less than 200,000/cmm, bone marrow aspiration to exclude leukemia is indicated. A sudden, rapid drop in the platelet count, especially with pancytopenia, and a fall in the ESR may indicate the development of macrophage activation syndrome (MAS), which is a dreaded complication of SJIA.
(f) Hyperferritinemia with serum ferritin levels typically >1000 (even ≥50,000 ng/mL) is also common in children with active SJIA. A sudden rise in the serum ferritin level occurs during MAS, and a ferritin/ESR ratio of >80 has been proposed as a biomarker of MAS.
(g) Elevation of cytokines IL-6 and specifically IL-18.
(h) Low-grade D-dimer positivity. Markedly elevated levels suggest the onset of MAS.
(i) Altered liver enzymes with increased levels of aspartate aminotransferase (AST) and alanine aminotransferase (ALT), hypoalbuminemia, and increased globulin levels. Markedly elevated hepatic enzymes, prolonged clotting times, should prompt immediate consideration of MAS.

Urinalysis is typically normal and hematuria or significant proteinuria suggest another diagnosis, such as systemic lupus erythematosus. Antinuclear antibodies (ANA) and rheumatoid factor (RF) are negative. Some chronic infectious processes, such as subacute bacterial endocarditis, can cause unexplained fevers and a positive RF.

Laboratory tests revealed no anti-nuclear antibodies, rheumatoid factor was negative, and serum ferritin level was elevated (4350 ng/mL). Repeated clinical examination failed to demonstrate arthritis. In view of the inconclusive clinical picture, a fludeoxyglucose-18 (FDG) positron emission tomography (PET) scan/CT scan was performed, in which both knees, and ankles showed mildly elevated uptake, suggesting synovitis. The images also revealed elevated metabolic activity diffusely in the spleen, the red bone marrow, and some inguinal lymph nodes. This pattern of metabolic activity, without signs of malignancy, was suggestive of SJIA.

5. *What is the usefulness of FDG-PET/CT scans in making a diagnosis of SJIA?*

The FDG-PET/CT scan provides high-quality images along with detection of foci of increased intracellular glucose metabolism. FDG accumulates in malignant tissues as well as at the sites of infection and inflammation due to increased glycolytic activity of inflammatory cells. Its clinical applications are spreading from oncology to the diagnosis of a variety of chronic or occult infections and inflammatory conditions like sarcoidosis, spondylodiscitis, vasculitis, and rheumatoid arthritis. Mild to moderately increased uptake of FDG in the bone marrow, and spleen, is a common, nonspecific finding in patients with fever due to proliferation of immune cells causing an interleukin-dependent upregulation of glucose transporters. In SJIA, the FDG-PET/CT scan may reveal synovitis of multiple joints which clinically look normal. Markedly increased FDG uptake in the red bone marrow, enlarged lymph nodes and the spleen, also points toward SJIA. The FDG-PET/CT scan helps in ruling out occult infections and malignancy.

6. *What is the cause of SJIA?*

The etiopathogenesis of JIA is unclear. It is considered an auto-inflammatory disorder in which dysregulation of the innate immune system is caused by interactions between genetic factors and environmental exposures. The symp-

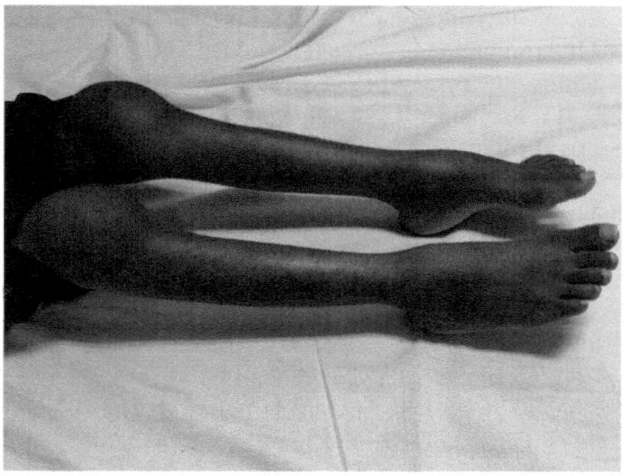

Fig. 15.3 Bilateral chronic arthritis of the knee and ankle joints. (Photo courtesy Dr. Mahesh Janardhanan)

toms result from pro-inflammatory cytokines like interleukin-1 (IL-1), IL-18, and IL-6 produced by the overstimulated innate immune system.

7. *What are the complications of SJIA?*

Macrophage activation syndrome (MAS) is a relatively common and potentially life-threatening complication which requires early recognition and immediate action. This is characterized by persistent fever, coagulopathy, pancytopenia, hepatitis, and extreme hyperferritinemia. If specific treatment is started early, the prognosis is good. In untreated patients, with SJIA, around 50% may develop other complications during the disease course which include severe articular damage due to erosive arthritis (Fig. 15.3), osteoporosis, growth retardation, pulmonary hypertension, amyloidosis, and complications caused by immunosuppressive drugs used in the treatment.

8. *How is SJIA treated?*

There is no cure for SJIA, but several drugs have been shown to reduce the severity of the symptoms and cause remission. Mild SJIA is treated initially with nonsteroidal anti-inflammatory drugs (NSAIDs) alone, while moderate to severe symptoms have been traditionally treated with corticosteroids. It is mandatory to rule out malignancy before starting steroids.

The disease-modifying antirheumatic drug (DMARD) methotrexate is added to steroid therapy for patients who fail to respond. However, in recent times, biologic DMARDs, such as interleukin (IL)-1 inhibitors (anakinra), are increasingly being used instead of steroids since they are highly effective, have fewer side effects, and prolonged corticosteroid therapy is associated with many complications.

15.2 Conclusion

On day 15 of illness, he was started on daily administration of naproxen. A marked decrease in fever spikes, pain, and inflammatory markers was seen within 3 days. He was discharged with advise to follow-up with the pediatric rheumatology team.

Learning Points

1. SJIA should be considered in the differential diagnosis of children with unexplained fever spikes, joint pain, rashes, and malaise.
2. In children <8 years of age, the signs of arthritis are subtle, and meticulous examination of the musculoskeletal system is an important component of evaluation of a young child with PUO.
3. In the presence of the typical quotidian fever pattern, SJIA should be considered even in the absence of arthritis and rashes which may not be evident early in the course of the disease.
4. The rash of SJIA is evanescent and may be difficult to see in darker-skinned individuals. Thus, careful inspection of the skin during the fever spike is important when SJIA is suspected.
5. Polymorphonuclear leucocytosis, markedly raised ESR and CRP with no evidence of infection, and hyperferritinemia are important clues.
6. In children presenting PUO without overt arthritis, FDG-PET/CT imaging is useful in identifying the sources of

inflammation as well as ruling out the differentials.
7. Macrophage activation syndrome (MAS) is a potentially life-threatening complication requiring early recognition and immediate treatment.
8. Early referral to a pediatric rheumatologist helps in making a diagnosis and initiating appropriate therapy early, thus limiting articular damage.

Suggested Readings

Grevich S, Shenoi S. Update on the management of systemic juvenile idiopathic arthritis and role of IL-1 and IL-6 inhibition. Adolesc Health Med Ther. 2017;8:125. https://doi.org/10.2147/AHMT.S109495.

Lee JJY, Schneider R. Systemic juvenile idiopathic arthritis. Pediatr Clin N Am. 2018;65(4):691–709. https://doi.org/10.1016/j.pcl.2018.04.005.

Sahba S, Huurnink A, Van den Berg JM, Tuitert B, Vastert SJ, Ten Tusscher GW. Systemic juvenile idiopathic arthritis in two children; case report on clinical course, challenges in diagnosis and the role of FDG-PET/CT-scan. Clin Case Rep. 2022;10:e05900. https://doi.org/10.1002/ccr3.5900.

Schönau V, Vogel K, Englbrecht M, et al. The value of 18F-FDG-PET/CT in identifying the cause of fever of unknown origin (FUO) and inflammation of unknown origin (IUO): data from a prospective study. Ann Rheum Dis. 2018;77(1):70–7. https://doi.org/10.1136/annrheumdis-2017-211687.

Torreggiani S, Filocamo G, Esposito S. Recurrent fever in children. Int J Mol Sci. 2016;17(4):448. https://doi.org/10.3390/ijms17040448.

Inflammatory Bowel Disease 16

Contents

> **Key Messages**
> Inflammatory bowel disease should be considered in the differential diagnosis of prolonged fever, fatigue, and abdominal pain, especially with loss of weight. Endoscopic evaluation of the GI tract with histopathologic examination of biopsies from the affected areas help in making the diagnosis.

16.1 Case Discussion

A 15-year-old adolescent boy presented with insidious onset, low-grade fever on and off for 1 month, with the maximum temperature recorded being 100.6 °F. He had easy fatigability and intermittent abdominal pain . Three weeks ago, he had crampy abdominal pain with semi-solid stools mixed with blood 3–4 times daily. The stools were not foul smelling, or greasy at any time. There was no vomiting. He was passing urine adequately. He was treated sequentially with oral cefixime and metronidazole. The loose stools with blood subsided within a week, but intermittent abdominal pain and fever persisted. There was a history of reduced activity, poor appetite, and weight loss. There was no past history of similar problems or recurrent infections. There was no history of any skin lesions or joint involvement.

On examination, he was very pale with mild pitting pedal edema. His body temperature was 100.4 °F, other vital signs were normal, and there were no signs of dehydration. There was no significant lymphadenopathy. He had moderate wasting. Head to foot examination revealed no abnormality. On abdominal examination, there was mild diffuse tenderness. There was no free fluid. Anal and perianal regions were normal.

1. *What are the clinical possibilities in this child with fever, fatigue, weight loss, and gastrointestinal symptoms?*

One should first consider the possibilities of gastrointestinal (GI) infections and systemic infections with GI involvement. Protozoal infec-

P. Venkat Ramanan, R. Padmanabhan, *Fever in Children*,
https://doi.org/10.1007/978-981-97-9967-1_16

tions like intestinal amebiasis can present with prolonged diarrhea with or without blood, abdominal pain, fever, and weight loss spanning from weeks to months. Intestinal tuberculosis (ITB) should always be considered in low- and middle-income countries (LMICs). A triad of abdominal pain, fever, and weight loss is suggestive of abdominal tuberculosis (TB) in children. A high index of suspicion is required to diagnose abdominal TB. History of contact with an active TB patient must always be elicited.

The boy was admitted for further evaluation. Blood investigations revealed a low Hb level of 4.7 g/dL; total and differential leukocyte counts were normal; and the platelet count was 5,20,000/cmm. Blood and urine culture showed no growth. Fresh stool examination repeated twice revealed WBCs and a few RBCs and there were no parasites. Erythrocyte sedimentation rate (ESR) was 56 mm/h, and liver enzymes and bilirubin levels were normal. Serum albumin was 2.8 g/dL. The Mantoux test was negative, and chest X-ray was normal. In view of all the tests for TB being negative, ITB was considered less likely.

2. *With common infections being ruled out, what are the other possibilities in this child?*

In an adolescent presenting with fever and gastrointestinal (GI) symptoms such as abdominal pain and diarrhea, other possibilities are immunodeficiencies and inflammatory conditions involving GI tract and rarely primary GI malignancies.

(a) Acquired immunodeficiency syndrome (AIDS) can present with loss of weight, diarrhea, and fever due to intestinal involvement. The GI manifestations in HIV infection may be due to cytomegalovirus (CMV), tuberculosis infection, or intestinal lymphoma.
(b) Inflammatory bowel disease (IBD) also requires consideration in view of fever, fatigue, loss of weight, and GI symptoms in this child.
(c) Among the primary malignancies of the GI tract in children, non-Hodgkin lymphoma (NHL) remains the most common. The most common presenting symptom of intestinal NHL is abdominal pain, followed by abdominal distension, vomiting, constipation, diarrhea, and intestinal obstruction.

HIV status was negative. In view of severe anemia, stool was tested for occult blood which was found to be positive. He was given a packed cell transfusion. In view of the persistent abdominal pain, wasting, low serum albumin levels, and occult blood in stools, the possibility of inflammatory bowel disease (IBD) was considered.

3. *What is inflammatory bowel disease (IBD)?*

Inflammatory bowel disease (IBD) is a chronic, idiopathic inflammatory disease of the gastrointestinal tract with a typical remitting and relapsing course. Crohn's disease (CD) and ulcerative colitis (UC) are the two major forms of IBD.

Crohn's disease involves the entire GI tract and perianal region (pan-enteric), while UC is typically confined to the colon. In CD, there are segments with inflammation alternating with normal areas (skipped lesions), strictures, and fistulas. Ileocolonic involvement is the most common presentation. There is inflammation involving all the layers of the bowel wall (transmural). The presence of granulomas in biopsy helps in differentiating CD from UC.

Ulcerative colitis is characterized by continuous inflammation of the rectum with proximal extension in the form of left-sided colitis, or pancolitis. Pancolitis is most common in children.

The usual age of presentation for both ulcerative colitis and Crohn's disease is between 15 and 30 years, although IBD can present at any age. The overall incidence of pediatric-onset IBD has been increasing over time. The incidence and prevalence of Crohn's disease and ulcerative colitis appear to be lower in Asia and the Middle East; but, in some newly industrialized countries in Africa, Asia, and South America, the incidence of IBD has been rising.

4. *When should the possibility of IBD be considered in the differential diagnosis of prolonged fever?*

The possibility of IBD should be considered in any child with prolonged fever, GI symptoms (diarrhea, rectal bleeding, and abdominal pain), and constitutional symptoms like fatigue, and weight loss. Clinical examination of abdomen is usually nonspecific other than abdominal tenderness. Extra-intestinal manifestations may be present in the form of arthritis, oral ulcers, clubbing, skin lesions such as erythema nodosum or pyoderma gangrenosum, uveitis, and hepatic involvement (primary sclerosing cholangitis and autoimmune hepatitis). Sometimes, extra-intestinal involvement is more prominent than intestinal symptoms. Rarely, IBD can present with sparse or absent gastrointestinal tract symptoms. Older children are more likely to present with abdominal pain, weight loss, and fever, in addition to GI bleeding, while young children typically present with only rectal bleeding.

5. *What investigations would help in establishing the diagnosis of IBD?*

Preliminary laboratory investigations may reveal anemia, thrombocytosis, raised ESR and CRP, and low serum albumin in IBD. Stool has to be examined for intestinal parasites such as *Entamoeba histolytica.* HIV infection must be ruled out. Calprotectin is a cytosolic protein complex derived from neutrophils, and fecal calprotectin levels increase with intestinal inflammation in IBD. When the fecal calprotectin levels are normal (<50 mg/g), the diagnosis of IBD can be ruled out with confidence. It has poor specificity and may be raised in other bacterial, *Helicobacter pylori*, and parasitic GI infections prevalent in developing countries.

A thorough assessment of the GI tract with upper and lower endoscopy and imaging (magnetic resonance (MR)/computed tomography (CT) enterography/ conventional fluoroscopy) is required. Biopsies from affected and unaffected areas of intestine are essential.

In CD, endoscopy reveals deep, irregular, serpiginous, longitudinal ulcers with normal intervening mucosa with involvement of ileum and sparing of rectum. The deep ulcers with a longitudinal array create a cobblestone appearance. Sparing of the rectum and occurrence of perianal disease, strictures, and fistulas suggest CD. In UC, diffuse, continuous superficial ulcers are seen which are friable with loss of vascular pattern. Rectal involvement and ileal sparing are characteristic. Biopsy of the affected region reveals non-caseating granuloma in CD.

Magnetic resonance enterography was done which revealed mural thickening of the entire large intestine and mild mural enhancement of the jejunum. Upper GI endoscopy (UGIE) and colonoscopy with terminal ileoscopy were done. UGIE revealed inflammation of the stomach lining, specifically in the body (corpus) of the stomach (corpus gastritis) and biopsy was taken. Colonoscopy revealed erythema with multiple aphthous ulcers throughout colon–pancolitis (Fig. 16.1). Multiple biopsies were taken. Biopsy from colon showed features of Crohn's disease (CD) (Fig. 16.2a, b).

6. *Can IBD present as pyrexia of unknown origin (PUO)?*

Fever is seen in about 14% of children with pediatric Crohn's disease. It is usually associated with gastrointestinal symptoms. Rarely, IBD can present with sparse or absent gastrointestinal tract symptoms. Diagnosis is made in such a situation with the help of imaging studies done for PUO workup, followed by colonoscopy and biopsy.

7. *What is the etiopathogenesis of IBD?*

Though the exact etiology of IBD is not known, genetic factors, intestinal microbiota, dietary factors, and immunological factors appear to have a role. Genetics is a very important risk factor for IBD, and up to 19–41% of children in the West may have an affected family member with IBD. Having a first-degree relative with IBD increases the risk to about 30-fold.

High dietary fiber consumption, higher intake of omega-3 fatty acids, lower intake of omega-6 fatty acids, and higher vitamin D intake are associated with lower frequency of IBD, while a high fat intake is correlated with increased risk of IBD. Smoking is

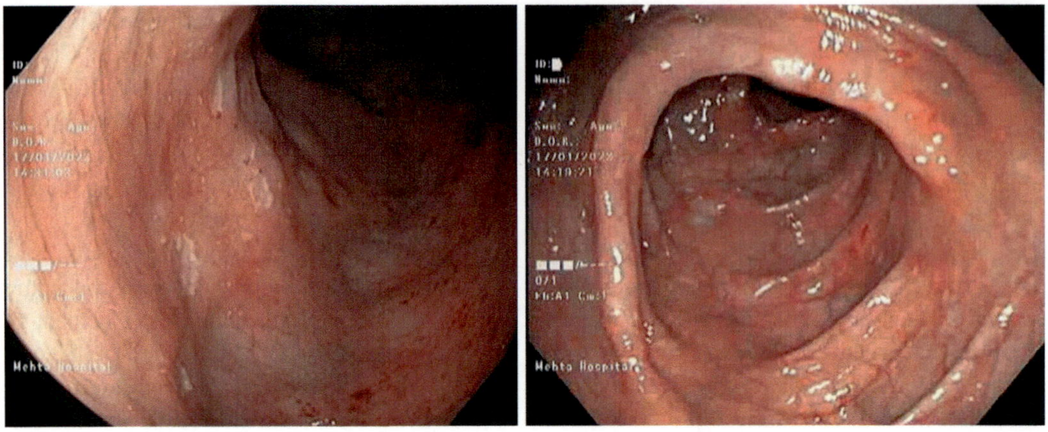

Fig. 16.1 Extensive aphthous ulcers on colonoscopy. (Picture courtesy: Dr. Sumathi Bavanandam, Pediatric gastroenterologist)

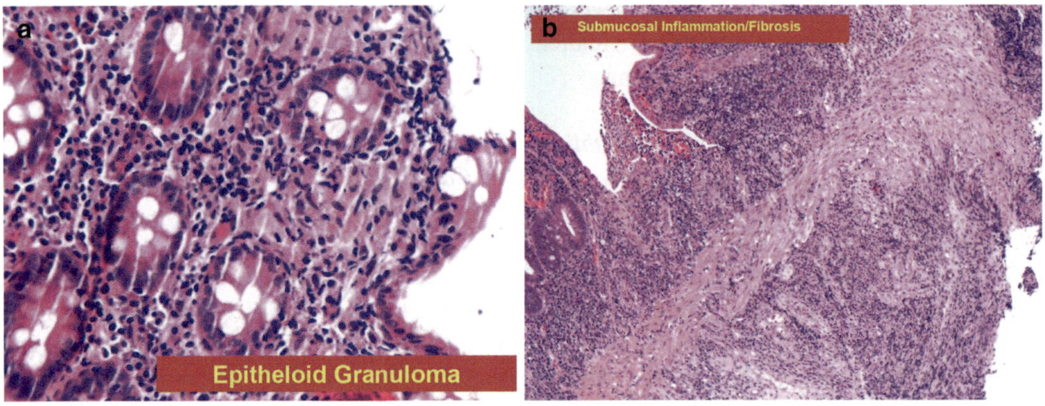

Fig. 16.2 (**a**) Non-caseating granulomas in biopsy. (**b**) Submucosal inflammation and fibrosis. (Picture courtesy: Dr. Sumathi Bavanandam, Pediatric gastroenterologist)

identified as a risk factor for Crohn's disease and its complications (strictures, fistula, and need for surgery) but not for ulcerative colitis.

8. *What are the clinical features of Crohn's disease and ulcerative colitis?*

In IBD, the clinical features depend upon the location of disease activity in the GI tract and the extent of the disease. Abdominal pain is the most frequent problem in pediatric Crohn's disease followed by diarrhea with or without blood, and growth failure which can manifest as weight loss/reduced weight gain or impaired height. Prolonged intermittent fever may be present. Perianal abnormalities such as fistulae, anal skin tags, or fissures are common in CD. Pubertal delay and malabsorption causing features of iron, vitamin D, and B12 deficiency may occur. The disease activity is assessed by Pediatric Crohn's disease activity index (PCDAI), which is based on the following parameters. Each of these have a score of 0, 5, or 10 depending on the severity.

(a) History: abdominal pain, number of stools per day, patient functioning.
(b) Examination: weight loss, height (at diagnosis/follow-up height velocity), abdomen (tenderness), perirectal disease, extra-intestinal manifestations.
(c) Laboratory: hematocrit, ESR, serum albumin.

A total score of 0 to 10 denotes inactive disease, 11 to 30 mild disease activity, and over 30 moderate to severe disease activity.

Children with UC present with diarrhea frequently containing blood, weakness, anemia, abdominal pain, and sometimes weight loss. More fulminant presentation is characterized by severe abdominal pain, frank bleeding per rectum, tenesmus, fever, leukocytosis, and hypoalbuminemia.

Similar to PCDAI, a pediatric UC activity index (PUCAI) has been developed to assess the activity of the disease. Scores are given for the following symptoms: (1) abdominal pain, (2) rectal bleeding, (3) stool consistency, (4) stool frequency, (5) nocturnal stools, and (6) activity level. Of these components, rectal bleeding has been given the maximum score.

9. *Does clinical presentation of IBD in children differ from that in adults?*

Children with IBD are at a higher risk for a more severe course of the disease and intestinal complications compared with adult-onset IBD. Pediatric IBD (PIBD) often interferes with growth and development. Early onset IBD (EOIBD) has a more aggressive clinical presentation and there are two subsets: very early onset IBD (VEOIBD) in children younger than 6 years and infantile onset in children less than 2 years. The disease commonly presents with colonic involvement and frank rectal bleeding. Distinguishing between UC and CD may be more difficult in this age group. They require immunologic evaluation and genetic sequencing for monogenic forms of IBD. They may require alternative therapies to the standard adult phenotype IBD.

10. *How does one differentiate between Crohn's disease and intestinal TB (ITB)?*

Intestinal tuberculosis is a close differential diagnosis of CD in both developing and developed countries. The differentiating features between CD and ITB are as follows:

(a) Colonoscopic appearance: In CD there are longitudinal ulcers, aphthous ulcers, a cobblestone pattern, and anorectal lesions, while in ITB there are circular transverse ulcers, patulous ileocecal valve, pseudo polyps, and the absence of transmural cracks and fissures.
(b) Other supportive evidence for ITB: Contact history of TB, Mantoux positivity, ascites with lymphocytes in ascitic fluid, necrotic, calcified abdominal lymph nodes in CT abdomen, and evidence of disseminated TB in other organs such as lung and CNS.
(c) Biopsy: HPE shows caseating large granulomas in ITB, and non-caseating granulomas are seen in IBD. The presence of granulomas in lymph nodes in the absence of granulomatous lesions in the intestine may also help in identifying ITB.
(d) Microbiology: Tissue sample showing acid -fast bacilli on microscopy, a positive cartridge -based nucleic acid amplification test (CBNAAT), or culture positivity clinches the diagnosis of TB.

When ITB cannot be ruled out, a trial of 8–12 weeks of antitubercular therapy is recommended by experts in developing countries.

11. *What is the management of Crohn's disease?*

The components of treatment in IBD are induction therapy, maintenance therapy, surgery, nutritional therapy, growth monitoring, and psychosocial support. While the primary objective is induction and maintenance of remission, careful monitoring of the impact of the disease and various interventions to optimize the growth and development are also important in children. For mild CD (involving only the terminal ileum and/or colon and no complications), aminosalicylates such as mesalamine are sometimes used for induction and maintenance therapy. Though they have low toxicity, their efficacy is questionable. Hence, close follow-up is required to confirm mucosal healing.

Induction therapy: Systemic steroids like prednisolone are used for induction therapy in moderate to severe CD in doses of 1 to 1.5 mg/kg and tapered over 8 to 12 weeks. In Western countries, anti-tumor necrosis factor (anti-TNF) antibodies such as infliximab or adalimumab are preferred for both induction and maintenance in moderate to severe CD and in steroid-unresponsive disease. Exclusive enteral nutrition (EEN) is also employed for induction in selected cases.

Maintenance therapy: Immunomodulators such as thiopurines (6-mercaptopurine [6-MP] or azathioprine [AZA]) and methotrexate (MTX) are used.

Before starting immunosuppressive drugs, the child should be evaluated for latent TB infection using tuberculin skin testing or interferon-gamma release assay.

Surgery in CD is indicated for those who do not respond to medical treatment or those developing complications such as abscess, fistula, perforation, hemorrhage, obstruction, or stricture. Ileal resection with partial colectomy and re-anastomosis or rarely subtotal/total colectomy, and strictureplasty are the type of surgeries that may be done.

12. *How is ulcerative colitis managed?*

For mild colitis (less than four stools, no significant abdominal pain, anemia, or fever), treatment is initiated with oral 5-ASA (mesalamine) or sulfasalazine.

For moderate colitis (more than four bloody stools per day, intermittent abdominal pain, but no tenesmus or fever), oral steroids such as prednisolone are started.

In those who cannot be weaned from steroids (steroid-dependent): Anti-TNF antibodies such as infliximab, adalimumab, or an immunomodulator such as 6-MP or azathioprine are recommended.

16.2 Conclusion

The child was started on steroids and mesalamine along with nutritional support. After 4 weeks, the steroids were tapered and stopped after 12 weeks, and the child was continued on azathioprine maintenance . He has responded well with reduction of GI symptoms and weight gain. He is on regular follow-up.

Acknowledgments We thank Dr. Sumathi Bavanandam, Professor of Gastroenterology at Stanley Medical College, Chennai for her role in managing the case and providing the colonoscopy and biopsy pictures.

Learning Points

1. In a child presenting with prolonged fever, fatigue, and abdominal pain, the possibility of inflammatory bowel disease (IBD) should be considered.
2. IBD is a chronic, idiopathic inflammatory disease of the gastrointestinal tract with a typical remitting and relapsing course.
3. Crohn's disease (CD) and ulcerative colitis (UC) are the two major forms of IBD, and the overall incidence of pediatric-onset IBD has been increasing over time.
4. Genetic factors, intestinal microbiota, dietary factors, and immunological factors appear to play a role in the evolution of IBD.
5. The usual age of presentation for IBD is between 15 and 30 years, although it can present at any age.
6. Crohn's disease may involve any part of the GI tract (ileocolonic being the most common). Inflammation of all layers of the bowel wall (transmural), segmental involvement alternating with normal areas known as skipped lesions, strictures, and fistulas may be seen.
7. Ulcerative colitis is typically confined to the colon with inflammation of the rectum with proximal extension.
8. Abdominal pain is the most frequent presentation in pediatric Crohn's disease followed by diarrhea with or without blood, growth failure, pubertal delay, prolonged fever, perianal fistulae or fissures, and anal skin tags.

9. UC presents with diarrhea, frequently containing blood, frank bleeding per rectum, tenesmus, fever, weakness, anemia, abdominal pain, and sometimes weight loss.
10. Extra-intestinal manifestations involving skin, joints, eyes, and liver may be seen in IBD.
11. The diagnosis of IBD is established by endoscopic evaluation with histopathologic examination of biopsies from the affected areas and imaging.
12. The presence of non-caseating granulomas in biopsy helps in differentiating CD from UC and also from intestinal TB.
13. IBD treatment involves induction and maintenance therapy, surgery, nutritional therapy, growth monitoring, and psychosocial support.
14. Steroids, biologicals such as anti-tumor necrosis factor antibodies (infliximab or adalimumab), immunomodulators such as azathioprine and methotrexate, and aminosalicylates such as mesalamine are the drugs used for CD and UC.

Suggested Readings

Bouhuys M, Lexmond WS, van Rheenen PF. Pediatric inflammatory bowel disease. Pediatrics. 2023;151(1):e2022058037. https://doi.org/10.1542/peds.2022-058037.

Gupta N, Bostrom AG, Kirschner BS, et al. Presentation and disease course in early-compared to later-onset pediatric Crohn's disease. Am J Gastroenterol. 2008;103(08):2092–8.

Kedia S, Das P, Madhusudhan KS, Dattagupta S, Sharma R, Sahni P, et al. Differentiating Crohn's disease from intestinal tuberculosis. World J Gastroenterol. 2019;25:418–32.

Kapoor A, Bhatia V, Sibal A. Pediatric inflammatory bowel disease. Indian Pediatr. 2016;53:993–1002.

Moon JS. Clinical aspects and treatments for pediatric inflammatory bowel diseases. Pediatr Gastroenterol Hepatol Nutr. 2019;22(1):50–6. https://doi.org/10.5223/pghn.2019.22.1.50.

Snapper SB. Very-early-onset inflammatory bowel disease. Gastroenterol Hepatol. 2015;11(08):554–6.

Yachha SK, Sarma MS. Inflammatory bowel disease. In: IAP recent advances in pediatrics. 1st ed. New Delhi: Jaypee Brothers Medical; 2020. p. 249–62.

17 Lymphoma

Contents

> **Key Messages**
> Mediastinal masses in childhood are usually malignant, and the most common malignancy is lymphoma. A chest radiograph is one of the first-line investigations in the evaluation of children with PUO even when there are no respiratory symptoms.

17.1 Case Discussion

A 9-year-old boy, previously well, presented with a history of moderate -grade, intermittent fever for 11 days. He said he felt tired during the fever episodes and had stopped going to school. He had no localizing signs, loss of appetite, or weight. He had received all his childhood vaccines till 10 years of age. There was no significant travel history. He had one elder sister and none of the other members of his family had any illness.

Examination revealed a well-appearing boy with normal body mass index and normal vital signs. He had mild pallor without any significant lymphadenopathy or organomegaly. His systemic examination was normal.

Laboratory examinations revealed a hemoglobin level of 9.7 g/dL, with a white blood cell (WBC) count of 8500/c mm, a normal differential count, and a platelet count of 2.65 lacs/c mm. His C-reactive protein (CRP) was 31.03 mg/L and erythrocyte sedimentation rate (ESR) was 19 mm/h.

Chest X-ray (CXR) was taken.

1. *Is chest X-ray indicated in the evaluation of a child with PUO even when there is no cough or respiratory findings?*

A chest radiograph is one of the first -line investigations in the evaluation of children with PUO. Radiological features of infections, collagen vascular disease, or connective tissue disorder (CTD), as well as malignancy, can be recognized even when there are no clinical features related to the respiratory system. Pneumonia can be present without a cough. Features of tuberculosis (TB) may be seen in chest X-ray.

P. Venkat Ramanan, R. Padmanabhan, *Fever in Children*,
https://doi.org/10.1007/978-981-97-9967-1_17

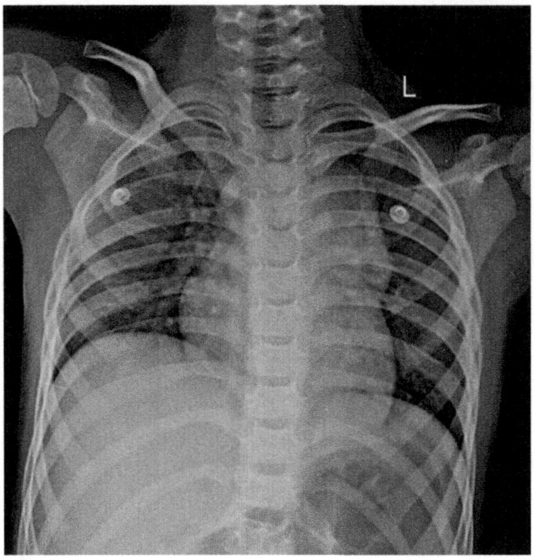

Fig. 17.1 Chest X-ray showing widening of left aspect of the mediastinum. (Photo courtesy Dr. Rishab T Ramesh)

CTD may show interstitial or pleural involvement, and malignancies in children may be seen as mediastinal masses.

The chest X-ray revealed a soft tissue opacity causing marked widening of the left aspect of the mediastinum with sharply defined lateral border and indistinct medial border (Fig. 17.1).

2. *What is the differential diagnosis in a child presenting with a mediastinal mass? Can childhood TB present like this?*

The causes of a mediastinal mass in childhood can be divided into congenital anomalies, infections, benign and malignant neoplasms, and normal variant (e.g., prominent thymus). In children, the normal thymus, which is the largest when the child is around 10 years of age, may be mistaken for a mediastinal mass. The differential diagnosis depends upon the anatomic compartment in which the mass is located.

Masses in the anterior mediastinum could be the thymus, retrosternal goiter, tumors arising from the parathyroid gland, pericardial cyst, teratoma, or lymphoma.

Middle mediastinal masses could be an enlarged lymph node, lymphoma, a vascular mass, or a bronchogenic cyst/tumor.

Posterior mediastinal masses could be an aortic aneurysm, a neurogenic tumor, a paraspinal abscess, a hiatal hernia, or a bronchogenic/esophageal tumor.

When there is fever with a mediastinal mass, the differential diagnosis includes infection and neoplasms. The infectious causes of lymph node enlargement in the mediastinum in children include TB, sarcoidosis, and histoplasmosis. TB presenting as an isolated mediastinal mass without parenchymal involvement is unusual.

A computed tomography and/or other imaging studies are often necessary to differentiate between these causes.

3. *What are the clinical presentations of a mediastinal mass?*

The mediastinal mass might be an incidental finding on imaging when the patient is being evaluated for an unrelated symptom or may cause symptoms due to compression or direct involvement of nearby structures. These include retrosternal chest pain, dysphagia, dyspnea, stridor, cough, superior vena caval - SVC compression with SVC syndrome, and hypotension (cardiac tamponade). Thus, a mediastinal mass may be misdiagnosed as asthma. Patients with large mediastinal masses who present with cardiorespiratory symptoms or radiographic evidence of tracheal obstruction are at increased risk of respiratory or cardiac arrest during general anesthesia or heavy sedation.

A CT scan of the chest revealed a soft -tissue homogenous mass in the anterior mediastinum, with smooth or lobulated margins. The possibility of lymphoma was considered.

4. *Is lymphoma a common cause of mediastinal mass in children*?

Seventy to seventy-five percent of mediastinal masses in childhood are malignant, and 45% of anterior mediastinal masses in children are lymphomas. Mediastinal lymphomas usually arise from either the thymus or lymph nodes, thus accounting for their predilection for the anterior and middle mediastinum.

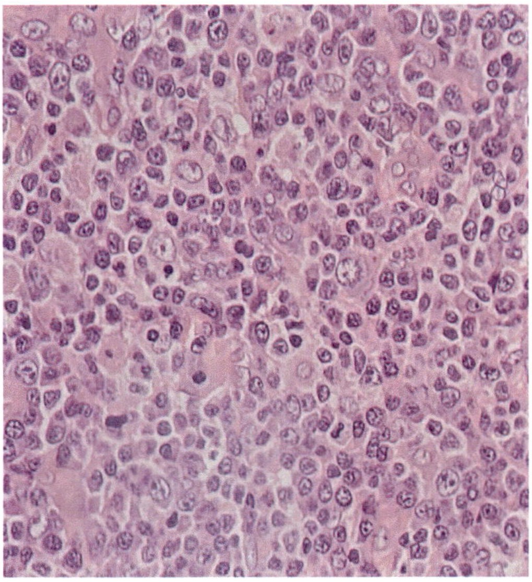

Fig. 17.2 Mediastinal biopsy, H&E stain 40 X showing monomorphous large atypical lymphoid cells. (Photo courtesy Dr. S. Sri Gayathri)

A CT -guided biopsy of the mediastinal mass was done and sent for histological examination and immunohistochemical analysis. Histologically, the lymph node architecture was completely replaced by monomorphous large atypical lymphoid cells, two to three times the size of mature lymphocytes, with scant cytoplasm and indented, angulated, and elongated nuclei (Fig. 17.2). The histological and immunohistochemical analyses confirmed a diagnosis of diffuse large B-cell lymphoma (B-LBL).

5. *What is a lymphoma? How does non-Hodgkin lymphoma (NHL) differ from Hodgkin lymphoma (HL)?*

Lymphoma is a group of malignant neoplasms derived from lymphocytes. Non-Hodgkin lymphoma (NHL) and Hodgkin lymphoma (HL) are the two main categories of lymphomas. NHL is more common in younger children, while Hodgkin lymphoma is more likely to affect older children and teens. HL usually begins in the upper body (neck, chest, or axilla), while NHL may arise from lymph nodes anywhere in the body. The clinical presentation and progression of HL is more predictable than non-Hodgkin lymphoma, making it easier to recognize and treat.

NHL is the fifth most common diagnosis of pediatric cancer in children under 15 years, and it accounts for approximately 7% of childhood cancers. Unlike in adults, most pediatric NHL cases are of high grade and aggressive. The median age at diagnosis is 10 years, and the incidence increases with age. The most common subtypes are Burkitt lymphoma, diffuse large B -cell lymphoma, lymphoblastic T -cell or B -cell lymphoma, and anaplastic large cell lymphoma.

6. *What are the various clinical presentations of NHL?*

NHL commonly presents as enlarged, nontender lymphadenopathy usually over 1–3 weeks. There may be clinical features due to the compression of surrounding structures and these depend on the areas of involvement. These could be new onset wheezing, retrosternal pain, stridor, dysphagia, respiratory distress, asymmetrical tonsils, or acute abdominal pain. Hepatomegaly and/or splenomegaly may be present in the advanced stage. A minority of patients have systemic complaints of fever, weight loss, or night sweats which are called B symptoms. The absence of these symptoms is classified as A.

For general pediatricians, an important point to note is that in a child presenting with symptoms of cough or wheezing for the first time, a CXR is essential before starting steroids for management of "asthma."

7. *What are the other investigations that help in suspecting a lymphoma?*

The complete blood count (CBC) may be normal. Extensive bone marrow infiltration, hypersplenism from splenic involvement, or blood loss from gastrointestinal tract involvement may cause anemia, thrombocytopenia, or leukopenia. Patients with rapidly proliferating tumors may have elevated uric acid, potassium, diminished renal function, or elevated level of serum lactate dehydrogenase. Initial imaging studies (e.g., ultrasound, radiographs, computed tomography) may demonstrate masses and/or lymphadenopathy in the neck, chest, or abdomen.

In addition, routine staging of pediatric NHL should include contrast enhanced computerized tomographic (CT) imaging of the neck, chest, abdomen, and pelvis. Positron emission tomography (PET)/CT scanning is more sensitive and specific than CT in the most common subtypes of NHL seen in children.

The diagnosis of NHL is based upon histopathological evaluation of the lymph node or extranodal mass. Subtypes of NHL are identified using histology, immunophenotype, and genetic studies.

8. *What are the life-threatening complications that a pediatrician should be aware of?*

NHL may present for the first time to a general pediatrician with an emergency complication that should be promptly recognized and treated. Depending on the location of the mass, the initial presentation may be acute airway obstruction, intestinal obstruction, intussusception, spinal cord compression, pericardial tamponade or lymphomatous meningitis, and/or CNS mass lesions. Another important complication is tumor lysis syndrome caused by the breakdown of large numbers of tumor cells. This releases large amounts of potassium, phosphate, and uric acid into the blood stream and deposition of uric acid and/or calcium phosphate crystals in renal tubules that can result in acute renal failure.

9. *How is NHL treated?*

A complete evaluation of patients with suspected NHL is mandatory before beginning treatment. The goal is to evaluate the extent of the disease, which in turn determines the clinical and pathologic stage, treatment, and, to a great extent, prognosis. Children with NHL should be treated in a comprehensive pediatric oncology center. A combination of chemotherapy is the primary modality used for the treatment of pediatric NHL. Unlike in adults, radiation therapy is not commonly used. Most children and adolescents with NHL have a good prognosis with current therapy.

17.2 Conclusion

The child was referred to the pediatric hematoncology unit where he received chemotherapy and responded well.

Learning Points

1. A chest radiograph is one of the first -line investigations in the evaluation of children with PUO even when there are no respiratory symptoms.
2. NHL commonly presents as enlarging, nontender lymphadenopathy usually over 1–3 weeks with symptoms due to the compression of surrounding structures.
3. A minority of lymphoma in children may present with fever, weight loss, or night sweats which are called B symptoms.
4. Seventy to 75% of mediastinal masses in childhood are malignant, and the most common malignancy is lymphoma.
5. The cough and wheeze caused by a mediastinal mass may be misdiagnosed as asthma. It is important to do a X-ray chest in children who present with wheeze for the first time before starting steroids.
6. NHL may also present for the first time to a general pediatrician with an emergency complication such as airway obstruction or SVC syndrome that should be promptly recognized and treated.
7. Pediatricians should promptly refer children and teenagers with a suspected NHL to a pediatric oncologist for evaluation and diagnosis.
8. The diagnosis of NHL is based upon histopathological evaluation of the lymph node or extranodal mass.

Suggested Readings

Piña-Oviedo S, Moran CA. Primary mediastinal nodal and extranodal non-Hodgkin lymphomas: current concepts, historical evolution, and useful diagnostic approach: part 2. Adv Anat Pathol. 2019;26(6):371–89. https://doi.org/10.1097/PAP.0000000000000248.

Verma S, Kalra K, Rastogi S, Sidhu HS. Clinical approach to childhood mediastinal tumors and management. Mediastinum. 2020;4:21. PMID: 35118289; PMCID: PMC8794350. https://doi.org/10.21037/med-19-82.

Melioidosis 18

Contents

Key Messages
PUO can be due to intra-abdominal abscesses, and they can occur even without the patient having any abdominal complaints at presentation. Melioidosis is being increasingly reported in India, and abscesses in internal organs, especially in the spleen (where they are often multifocal) and liver, are well -recognized features of melioidosis in children.

18.1 Case Discussion

An 8-year-old boy was brought with a history of high-grade fever for 2 weeks with loss of appetite and reduced activity. In the first week of fever, he had vomiting and mild epigastric pain. He was evaluated elsewhere as an outpatient and the available reports revealed a Hb level of 9.4 g/dL, a total leukocyte count (TLC) of 11,700 cells/mm^3 with a differential count of 62% polymorphs and 37% lymphocytes, a platelet count of 2.3 lakhs/mm^3, and a CRP of 5.6 mg/L. He had been treated for "typhoid fever" with oral cefixime for 1 week, but no blood culture reports were available. As high-grade fever continued, he was referred to our hospital. Vomiting had stopped but mild, intermittent abdominal pain continued. There was no history of any diarrhea, constipation, jaundice, rash, joint pain, or any other localizing symptoms. There was no history of contact with tuberculosis or consumption of unpasteurized milk. He had been immunized according to the national immunization schedule till 5 years of age.

On examination, he was underweight but well preserved. His vital signs were normal and he had pallor. There were no significant lymph nodes, rashes, or jaundice. Palpation of the abdomen revealed a liver of 3 cm below the right costal margin and a soft spleen, both being tender.

1. *What is the differential diagnosis of prolonged fever (>7 days) with hepatosplenomegaly?*

The common causes of prolonged fever with hepatosplenomegaly in children in the order of frequency are infectious diseases, connective

P. Venkat Ramanan, R. Padmanabhan, *Fever in Children*,
https://doi.org/10.1007/978-981-97-9967-1_18

tissue diseases, and neoplasms. The common generalized infections include enteric fever, malaria, disseminated tuberculosis, brucellosis, leptospirosis, and Epstein–Barr virus (EBV) infection. Fever with organomegaly can also be due to localized infections like hepatitis and intra-abdominal abscesses in the liver/spleen. Connective tissue disorders like juvenile idiopathic arthritis, systemic lupus erythematosus, and malignancies like leukemia and lymphoma can also cause fever with hepatosplenomegaly. A good history and thorough physical examination and sequential investigations will help in identifying the cause.

A clinical diagnosis of partially treated enteric fever was made. He was hospitalized for evaluation, and investigations revealed hypochromic microcytic anemia (Hb 7.9 g%), raised CRP level (214.1 mg/L), polymorphonuclear leukocytosis (total leucocyte count was 17,890/cu mm with 70% neutrophils), and an ESR of 32 mm first hour. He was started on IV antibiotics.

USG abdomen was done, and it showed an ill-defined hetero-echoic focal lesion in the right lobe of the liver (Fig. 18.1a). A few hypoechoic areas were noted within the center of the lesion suggestive of the liquefied component of an abscess (Fig. 18.1b).

In addition, an ill-defined hetero-echoic focal collection was noted in the lower pole of the spleen (Fig. 18.2a, b).

2. *What is the usefulness of abdominal imaging in a child presenting with prolonged fever? How do you decide on the choice of imaging?*

In a child with prolonged fever, abdominal imaging can provide clues to the cause of fever. It is useful in assessing the size and structure of the abdominal organs, mainly the liver and spleen. Hepatosplenomegaly is seen in certain infections, autoimmune diseases, and malignancies. The echogenicity of the liver parenchyma can indicate the type of liver involvement. Ascites, intra-abdominal abscesses, and enlarged abdominal lymph nodes suggestive of systemic infection/malignancies can be visualized. Imaging can also identify structural abnormalities and signs of inflammation in the stomach, intestines, and blood vessels that could be the cause of fever.

The choice of the imaging modality required depends on the most likely underlying conditions and the specific information required. USG is the initial modality of choice as it is noninvasive, cost-effective, and safe (no radiation exposure),

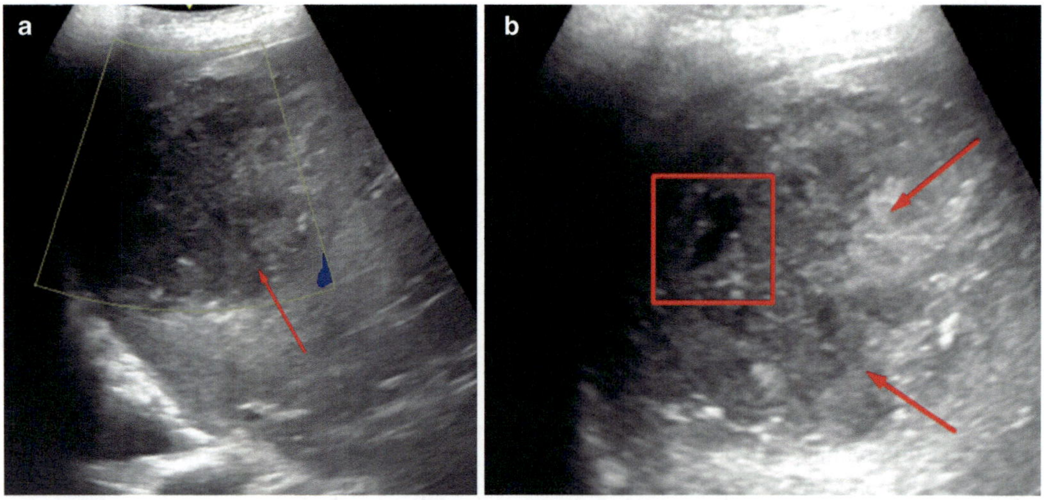

Fig. 18.1 (**a**) Abdominal USG showing an ill-defined hetero-echoic lesion in the right lobe of the liver with no evidence of internal vascularity. (Images courtesy Dr. Rishab Ramesh). (**b**) Hypoechoic areas within the center of the lesion. (Images courtesy Dr. Rishab Ramesh)

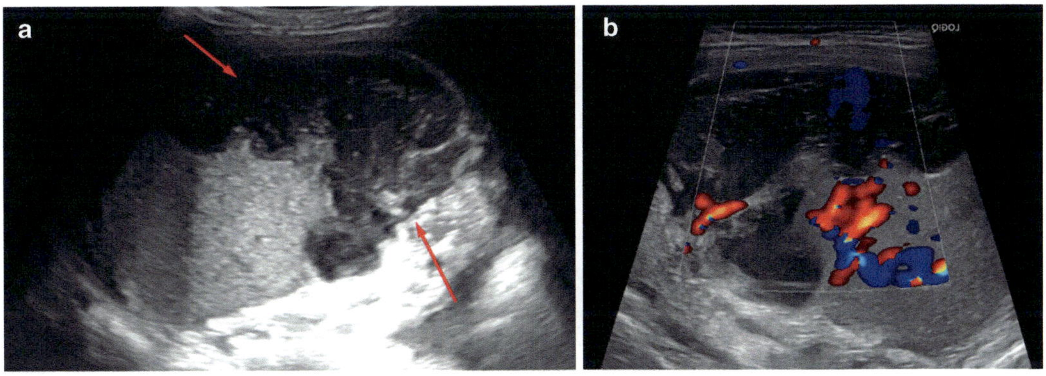

Fig. 18.2 (**a** and **b**) Abdominal USG showing ill-defined hetero-echoic collection in the lower pole of the spleen measured with peripheral increased vascularity. (Images courtesy Dr. Rishab Ramesh)

especially in pediatric patients. However, the deeper structures or organs may be obscured by bowel gas. It may miss subtle abnormalities and small lesions. A CT provides a more detailed imaging of organs and can detect small lesions, abscesses, or vascular abnormalities that may not be visible on USG. CT is quicker than prolonged ultrasound examinations. However, it involves exposure to ionizing radiation, and if a contrast-enhanced CT (CECT) is needed there is a small risk of allergic reactions and renal injury. So a CT is reserved for situations in which the ultrasound is inconclusive or it reveals a pathology that requires further evaluation.

3. *What are the causes of hetero-echoic focal lesions in the liver and spleen?*

Hetero-echoic focal lesions in the liver and spleen on ultrasound can be seen in abscesses, tumors (lymphangioma, hemangioma), and cysts (pseudocysts, hydatid cysts). Cysts appear as fluid collections without surrounding stranding or hyperemia, while tumors have a solid appearance and sometimes areas of calcification. Necrosis/ bleeding into a tumor may sometimes simulate the fluid-filled appearance of an abscess. In this child, the ultrasound features with the history of fever suggested abscesses. The radiologists suggested a CT scan of the abdomen for better characterization and to look for evidence of rupture as well as communications with surrounding structures like the biliary tree/diaphragm which are better visualized on a cross section.

The CT scan of the abdomen revealed an enlarged liver measuring 18 cm with a well-defined peripherally located thin-walled hypodense cystic lesion of size 8.0 × 6.7 × 7.0 cm (AP × CC × TR) involving segments VII and VIII of the right lobe of liver. On contrast administration, the lesion showed peripheral enhancement with a central non-enhancing area, suggestive of necrotic changes (Fig. 18.3a). A few discrete, thin, incomplete septa were noted within.

The spleen was mildly enlarged, and an ill-defined peripherally enhancing hypodense collection at the hilum coalescing with a similar subcapsular collection at the lower pole, collectively measuring 6.0 × 5.8 × 5.8 cm (volume ~ 100 cc) was observed. A few thick internal septations were noted (Fig. 18.3b, c).

4. *When should an intra-abdominal abscess be suspected as a cause of PUO?*

PUO can be due to intra-abdominal abscesses, which include liver, subdiaphragmatic, perinephric, splenic and pelvic abscesses, and they can occur without the patient having any abdominal complaints at presentation. The possibility of an intra-abdominal abscess increases if the patient has a history of abdominal pain, prior intra-abdominal disease, or abdominal surgery. Pyogenic liver abscesses can present with tender hepatomegaly. Liver enzymes are usually nor-

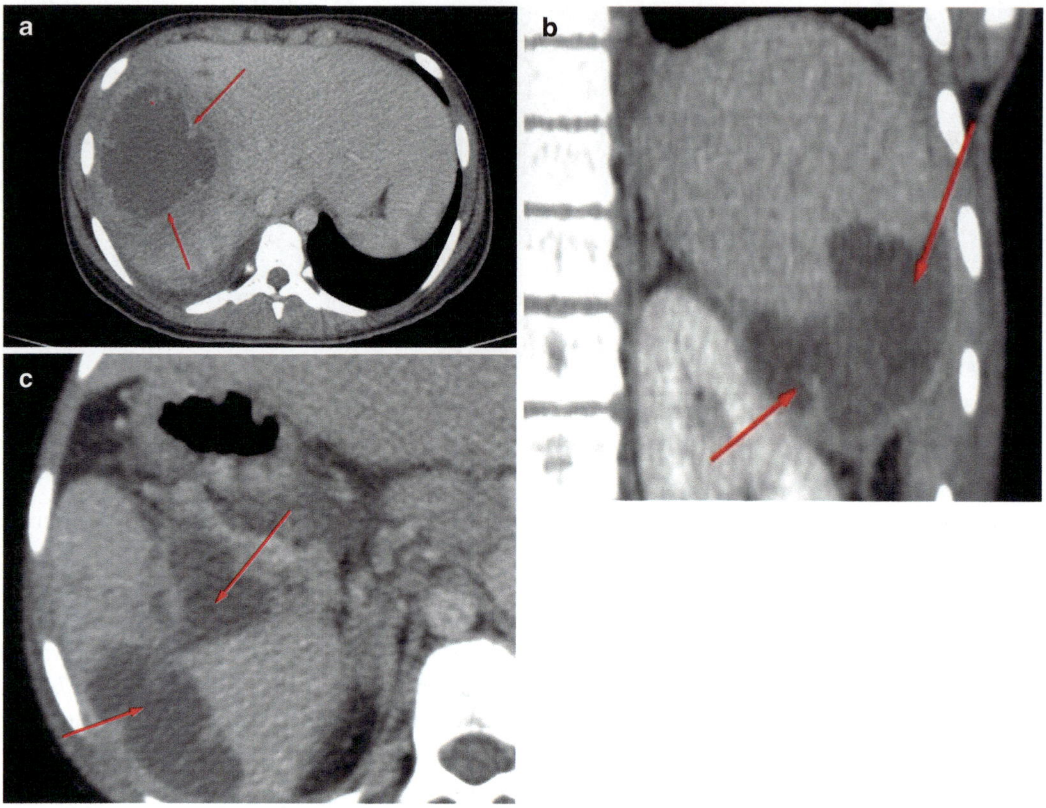

Fig. 18.3 (**a**) CECT of the abdomen showing a thin -walled hypodense cystic lesion in right lobe of the liver with peripheral enhancement on contrast. (Images courtesy Dr. Rishab Ramesh). (**b** and **c**) CECT of the abdomen showing mildly enlarged spleen with an ill-defined peripherally enhancing hypodense collection at the hilum coalescing with a similar subcapsular collection in the lower pole. (Images courtesy Dr. Rishab Ramesh)

mal, and blood culture is usually sterile. Imaging of the abdomen, typically with ultrasonography or CT, generally demonstrates intra-abdominal abscesses.

5. *What are the common causes of hepatic and splenic abscesses?*

Abscesses in the liver and spleen can occur due to hematogenous seeding from distant sites of infection or by spread from a contiguous focus like the biliary tree, pancreas, subphrenic abscess, or an infected bowel segment. Trauma and ischemia due to hemoglobinopathies are predisposing factors for splenic abscesses, and immunocompromised states are a risk factor for all abscesses. The microbiology of hepatic and splenic abscesses is highly variable. Depending upon the source of the abscess, common pathogens include *Staphylococcus aureus*, streptococci, *Salmonella*, *Klebsiella*, *Escherichia coli*, and anaerobes. Tuberculosis and parasitic infections such as amebiasis can also cause abscesses in the liver and spleen in children. The less commonly reported organisms include fungi like *Candida*, *Aspergillus*, and histoplasma and *Burkholderia pseudomallei*, which causes melioidosis.

6. *What is the management of liver/splenic abscess?*

In every case of liver/splenic abscess, pursuing a microbiological diagnosis is important. The abscess should be aspirated with CT or ultrasound-guidance. A purulent aspirate would suggest a pyogenic abscess. The aspirate should be sent for Gram stain and culture (both aerobic and anaerobic), and some material should be preserved in the laboratory for future testing, if needed. These tests include microscopy and culture for fungi and mycobacteria, antigen, or polymerase chain reaction (PCR) testing for *Entamoeba histolytica*, special stains for parasites, and 16S rRNA PCR testing for fastidious bacteria. If the aspirate is not purulent, biopsy material should be obtained and submitted for histopathology and cytology in addition to microbiology.

Antimicrobial therapy will be guided by the microbiology report. In cases of small abscesses, needle aspiration alone may be sufficient but larger abscess nccd a drainage. The material obtained from percutaneous drains should not be sent for culture since they are often contaminated with skin flora and environmental organisms and do not reliably guide antimicrobial therapy.

Both the abscesses were aspirated under USG guidance. The purulent material was obtained and sent for microbiological investigations. The pus culture was reported as *Burkholderia pseudomallei* sensitive to imipenem, ceftazidime, and cotrimoxazole.

7. *What is melioidosis?*

Melioidosis is a tropical infection caused by *Burkholderia pseudomallei*, a gram-negative bacillus that resides in soil and water. South Asia is estimated to have 44% of the global disease burden. The disease has also been reported in Southeast Asia, China, and Northern Australia. Among South Asian countries, Bangladesh and Sri Lanka are considered endemic. India has been reporting an increase in numbers of cases of melioidosis in recent years. Transmission occurs through percutaneous inoculation, inhalation, aspiration, and ingestion. Ingestion of contaminated water in endemic regions could explain the much higher rate of parotid and liver abscesses in parts of Southeast Asia. Unlike diabetes mellitus in adults, children with melioidosis usually do not have identifiable risk factors.

8. *What are the clinical features of melioidosis?*

Most infections with *B. pseudomallei* are asymptomatic or subclinical. The most common clinical manifestation of acute infection is pneumonia; other sites of infection include skin and soft tissue and the genitourinary tract. Bacteremic spread of the organism can result in abscess formation in virtually any site with clinical manifestations related to that site. Bacteremic patients can present with septic shock. Chronic infection may present as a nonhealing skin ulcer or abscess or may mimic pulmonary tuberculosis. *B. pseudomallei* infections are generally less severe in children compared with adults; they are more likely to present as skin infection and less likely to have bacteremia or pneumonia. In Southeast Asia, suppurative parotitis is a common presentation in childhood. Abscesses in internal organs are well recognized, especially in the spleen (where they are often multifocal), kidneys, prostate, and liver. Studies from Malaysia have shown that spleen is one of the most common affected organs in pediatric melioidosis. A study from Thailand has reported liver and/or spleen abscesses in 44% of cases (Chanvitan et al. 2019). Fevers, chills, and rigors with and without hypotension are common, but localizing symptoms are often absent. The less common sites of infection include bone and joint involvement and neurologic involvement.

9. *How is melioidosis diagnosed?*

Imaging tests like chest X -ray, CT scan, and MRI can reveal solid organ abscesses. Culture is the primary method of diagnosis. When melioidosis is suspected, blood and specimen from the site of infection such as sputum in lung infection, swab from the skin lesion, and pus/aspirate from abscesses should be sent for microbial examination and culture. A culture of *B. pseudomallei* from any clinical specimen is diagnostic for melioidosis because the bacterium is not part of the natural flora in any part of the human body. Blood culture has poor sensitivity. The organism is sometimes mistaken as *Pseudomonas* spp. in the laboratories and dismissed as a laboratory contaminant. A monoclonal antibody-based latex agglutination assay for *B. pseudomallei* is very useful for screening suspected colonies. Matrix-assisted laser desorption/ionization time of flight (MALDI-TOF) mass spectrometry has been used increasingly more frequently for the accurate identification of *B. pseudomallei.*

10. *How is melioidosis treated?*

Treatment of melioidosis comprises an acute phase in which ceftazidime or meropenem is given for 10 to 14 days by intravenous route. This is followed by the eradication phase during which oral trimethoprim–sulfamethoxazole or doxycycline is given for 3 to 6 months. Amoxicillin–clavulanate may be used as an alternative in pregnant women. Abscesses need to be drained either percutaneously or through an open procedure with concomitant recommended antibiotics.

18.2 Conclusion

The child was started on intravenous ceftazidime, and percutaneous pigtail catheters were inserted for drainage into both the abscess cavities. Fever spikes started reducing on day 4, and the child became afebrile on day 7 of IV ceftazidime. Repeat ultrasound on day 10 showed collapse of the abscess cavities. Hence, the catheters were removed. IV ceftazidime was given for a total period of 14 days after which he was discharged on oral trimethoprim–sulfamethoxazole. Repeat ultrasound after 3 months showed complete resolution of the abscesses. Hence, oral medication was stopped. On follow-up, he remained asymptomatic.

Learning Points

1. PUO can be due to intra-abdominal abscesses, and they can occur without the patient having any abdominal complaints at presentation.
2. The differential diagnoses for focal lesions of spleen and liver include cystic lesions, infective or inflammatory processes, and malignancies.
3. Melioidosis is a tropical infection caused by *B. pseudomallei*, a gram-negative bacillus that resides in soil and water of South and Southeast Asia. Hence, the residence and travel history are important in the workup of fever.
4. Transmission occurs through percutaneous inoculation, inhalation, aspiration, and ingestion.
5. The clinical features are diverse, with most of the reported cases presenting with pneumonia in adults and intra-abdominal abscess or parotid abscesses in children.
6. The diagnosis is established by culture of the organism from the blood, sputum, or pus obtained by aspiration of abscess.
7. India has been reporting an increase in number of cases of melioidosis in recent years, and the southern part of India is a new hotspot in the global map.
8. Melioidosis was thought to be a rare entity because of clinical ignorance as well as the organism being mistaken as *Pseudomonas* spp. in laboratories.
9. The treatment of melioidosis comprises two phases: acute phase—either ceftazidime or meropenem; and eradication phase— with cotrimoxazole, doxycycline, or amoxicillin–clavulanate.

Suggested Readings

https://wwwnc.cdc.gov/travel/yellowbook/2024/infections-diseases/melioidosis. Accessed 18 May 2024.

Mohapatra PR, Mishra B. Burden of melioidosis in India and South Asia: challenges and ways forward. Lancet Reg Health Southeast Asia. 2022;2:100004.

McLeod C, Morris PS, Bauert PA, et al. Clinical presentation and medical management of melioidosis in children: a 24-year prospective study in the Northern Territory of Australia and review of the literature. Clin Infect Dis. 2015;60:21.

Wiersinga WJ, Virk HS, Torres AG, Currie BJ, Peacock SJ, Dance DAB, Limmathurotsakul D. Melioidosis. Nat Rev Dis Primers. 2018;4:17107. PMID: 29388572; PMCID: PMC6456913. https://doi.org/10.1038/nrdp.2017.107.

19 Infective Endocarditis

Contents

Key Messages
Infective endocarditis may present as fever without a focus. Children with persistent *Staphylococcus aureus* bacteremia should be evaluated for metastatic infections including IE. In isolated right-sided IE, the cardiac murmur is usually faint or absent and embolization which occurs into the pulmonary circulation may mimic a respiratory tract infection.

19.1 Case Discussion

A 7-year-old boy presented with a history of fever for 10 days with occasional cough. The fever was low to moderate grade with a maximum temperature of 102.4 °F. It was sometimes associated with chills and body ache. He had no localizing symptoms. He had been hospitalized 1 week before the onset of fever with a diagnosis of severe dengue fever. He was in the pediatric intensive care unit (PICU) for 3 days, received intravenous (IV) fluids, and had recovered fully at the time of discharge. There was no other significant past medical or surgical history. He was fully immunized according to the national immunization schedule. There was no history of fever in the family, history of travel, or pets.

In the first week of fever, he was initially treated with oral amoxicillin for a presumed respiratory infection as there were no complaints suggestive of other systems involvement. When fever persisted, he was hospitalized elsewhere, and his investigations revealed a neutrophilic leucocytosis and an erythrocyte sedimentation rate (ESR) of 44 mm in the first hour. He was started on IV ceftriaxone to which fever responded initially. His cultures were sterile and other investigations were normal. As no conclusive diagnosis could be made and his fever returned after the initial response, he was referred to our hospital.

On examination, he was febrile with a temperature of 101.2 °F and was ill-appearing. His heart rate was 115/min and respiratory rate was 30/min. There was no respiratory distress. His general physical examination and systemic examination were normal.

P. Venkat Ramanan, R. Padmanabhan, *Fever in Children*,
https://doi.org/10.1007/978-981-97-9967-1_19

1. *What is the possible cause of fever a week after discharge in a child hospitalized in the PICU for severe dengue?*

When fever develops a week after discharge in a child who was hospitalized in the PICU for severe dengue, the following possibilities should be considered:

(a) A new community-acquired infection, bacterial or viral, unrelated to the previous episode of dengue.
(b) Immune-mediated mechanisms such as infection-triggered hemophagocytic lymphohistiocytosis (HLH).
(c) **Hospital-acquired infections (HAIs)**, especially after a stay in the PICU, bloodstream infection (sepsis), pneumonia, and urinary tract infection (UTIs) may develop.

The child was hospitalized for further evaluation. His initial investigations revealed a hemoglobin level of 9.6 g/dL, a WBC count of 24,000/cmm with 78% neutrophils, and a C-reactive protein level (CRP) of 12 mg/dL. The chest X-ray showed focal pulmonary infiltrates. The possibility of a bacterial infection was considered. Blood cultures were sent, and the child was started on intravenous injection ceftriaxone. The microbiology laboratory called 48 h later to report a growth of *Staphylococcus aureus* in the blood culture, and 24 h later, the antibiogram was released reporting as methicillin-resistant *Staphylococcus aureus* (MRSA).

2. *What is the treatment for MRSA bacteremia?*

Once the antimicrobial susceptibility is confirmed, vancomycin is the first-line treatment for MRSA. Depending on the patient's condition, other options that could be considered are linezolid, clindamycin, and ceftaroline. The duration of antibiotic therapy ranges from 2 to 6 weeks based on the extent of infection, response to treatment, presence of complications, and underlying medical conditions. Identification and management of the source of bacteremia is important. It may be an intra-abdominal or perianal abscess which was hitherto unnoticed. The management includes tackling the source such as drainage of abscesses, removal of indwelling devices (such as central venous catheters, CVCs), and surgical debridement of infected tissues. Strict infection control measures should be implemented to prevent the spread of MRSA to others. Repeat blood cultures should be obtained to assess for clearance of bacteremia. Factors such as the severity of illness, presence of underlying comorbidities, and response to treatment should be considered when determining the frequency of repeat blood cultures. In uncomplicated cases, repeat blood cultures may be obtained after 2–4 days of antibiotic therapy.

The child was started on IV vancomycin and supportive care. The fever continued unabated. Liver and kidney function tests showed no abnormalities. Serology for viruses (HIV, EBV, HBV, and HCV) and autoimmune markers (ANA, RF) which had been tested earlier were negative. Blood culture was repeated after 48 h of initiating antibiotics. Repeat culture also grew MRSA.

3. *What are the causes of persistent MRSA bacteremia despite treatment with adequate doses of appropriate antibiotics?*

Persistent bacteremia could be due to antibiotic resistance or inadequate source control including bacteremia complicated by infective endocarditis (IE), osteomyelitis, or occult infections.

The child was re-examined for any missed foci of infections. There were no clinical signs of skin/soft tissue infections or bone/joint infections. Repeated clinical examination of all systems did not reveal any new findings. The abdominal ultrasound was normal. A 2 D transthoracic echocardiography (ECHO) was performed to look for evidence of infective endocarditis.

4. *Is echocardiography (ECHO) indicated in every child with Staphylococcus bacteremia?*

In a child with *Staphylococcus aureus* bacteremia, echocardiography is indicated when bacteremia persists despite appropriate antibiotic therapy, or if there are recurrent episodes of bacteremia. It is also indicated if there is an underlying risk factor for IE such as a congenital or acquired heart disease, or there are clinical features of IE.

The ECHO revealed a vegetation of 1.1 cm × 0.9 cm attached to the anterior tricuspid valve (TV), and low-grade tricuspid regurgitation. Because of fever, persistent bacteremia, and ECHO findings, a definite diagnosis of native TV infective endocarditis (TVIE) was made using modified Duke criteria.

5. *What is IE and what are the causative organisms?*

Infective endocarditis is an infection of the endocardium, and it primarily involves the heart valves. Any event that leads to bacteremia can potentially predispose a child to develop infective endocarditis. In children, the main predisposing condition is a congenital heart disease. The structural lesions produce turbulent blood flow that might produce endocardial damage facilitating the development of a localized thrombotic reaction where a nidus of platelets and fibrin develops. When bacteremia occurs, the organisms adhere to this thrombotic area and a vegetation is formed comprising platelets, fibrin, microorganisms, and inflammatory cells. Organisms multiply, and the vegetations may break releasing septic emboli into the bloodstream. Occasionally, IE can involve a structurally normal heart also. These children have an increased risk of complications compared to those with a predisposing cardiac condition as a more aggressive pathogen causes the infection. Globally, *S. aureus* is the predominant cause of IE, especially in children without heart disease. *Streptococcus viridans* in the most common cause in those with an underlying heart disease.

6. *What are the clinical features of IE?*

The most common symptom is fever, seen in up to 90% of patients. In acute IE, fever may also be high grade and the course is fulminant. In subacute IE, which is more common, there is persistent low-grade fever which may be associated with malaise, joint pain, anorexia, and weight loss. On clinical examination, pallor and mild jaundice may be present. Though clubbing is described as a feature in subacute IE, it is rarely seen nowadays. Cardiac examination may show new or changing murmurs and acute heart failure due to valve damage. IE involves the left heart more commonly than the right and in left-sided IE, symptoms of systemic embolization may be present (glomerulonephritis, seizures, or cerebral infarction due to cerebral embolisms).

In right-sided IE, in 90% of cases, the tricuspid valve is involved; in the remaining, it is the pulmonic valve. The diagnosis of isolated right-sided IE is difficult because the symptoms are less obvious, the cardiac murmur is usually faint or absent, and embolization occurs into the pulmonary circulation which may mimic a respiratory tract infection. Most patients of TVIE have respiratory involvement at presentation. The risk factors for right-sided IE include indwelling catheters, immunocompromised states, congenital heart diseases, and intravenous drug injections.

7. *What are the criteria currently used for diagnosing IE?*

The modified Duke criteria are used to diagnose IE in children. Definite IE is defined as two major OR one major + three minor criteria, whereas possible IE requires one major + one minor OR three minor criteria. The major criteria are blood culture positive for a typical microorganism (i.e., *Staphylococcus aureus*, *Enterococcus*, *Streptococcus viridans*, and echocardiography findings such as valvular vegetation), and the minor criteria are the presence of a predisposing condition, fever, embolic phenomena, and immunologic phenomena (glomerulonephritis, Osler's nodes, Roth's spots, and rheumatoid factor).

8. *What are the investigations useful in diagnosing IE?*

Blood culture is the most important investigation in IE. Three sets of blood cultures (both aerobic and anaerobic culture bottles) should be sent when IE is suspected. The yield is higher with serial blood cultures (taking three samples at intervals of 1 h). Adequate volumes of blood should be processed and incubated for at least 5 days. Blood cultures may be sterile because of previous treatment with antibiotics, infections by slow-growing organisms, or inadequate microbiological techniques. With advances in microbiological diagnostic techniques, microbiological cause can be identified in 90% of cases. If no organism is cultured, if the child is stable, one could consider withholding antibiotics for 72 h and repeating the blood culture in suspected IE. When blood cultures are sterile, molecular techniques such as PCR, to detect bacterial DNA or the 16S subunit of bacterial ribosomes, should be considered. When symptoms (fever, inflammatory parameters in laboratory tests, and systemic inflammatory response) are persistent or recurrent, blood cultures should be repeated.

Transthoracic echocardiography should be performed in all suspected cases of IE. Features suggestive of IE include vegetations, abscesses, and a new dehiscence of a valvular prosthesis. In adults, transesophageal echocardiography has a greater sensitivity, but in children with a body weight < 60 kg, transthoracic echocardiography is comparable because of their better acoustic window. Other imaging techniques like cardiac magnetic resonance imaging, computed tomographic angiography, or positron emission tomography with computed tomography (PET-CT) are useful in children because congenital heart disease predisposes to TVIE which is poorly visualized on echocardiography, especially when a previous surgical correction has been performed.

Other investigations that support the diagnosis of IE include anemia (either hemolytic or anemia of chronic disease), elevated inflammatory markers (e.g., erythrocyte sedimentation rate [ESR], C-reactive protein [CRP], procalcitonin), and microscopic hematuria/red blood cell casts suggestive of glomerulonephritis. The chest radiograph may show nonspecific findings like cardiomegaly and focal pulmonary infiltrates in patients with pulmonary septic emboli.

9. *What is the treatment for IE?*

IE is treated with intravenous antibiotics. The choice and duration will depend on the causative microorganism and the susceptibility as per the antibiogram, and the patient's risk factors. MRSA IE is treated with vancomycin or daptomycin for 4–6 weeks. When antibiogram is not available, empirical antibiotic therapy need to be started as soon as possible. The usual regimen for an unknown organism is ampicillin + gentamicin + cloxacillin. In health-care-associated IE or if the child has a prosthetic valve, the choice would be vancomycin + gentamicin + rifampin to cover for MSSA and MRSA.

10. *How can IE be prevented?*

Currently, antibiotic prophylaxis is recommended only for patients with a few heart conditions (listed below) undergoing oral procedures in which manipulation of the dental mucosa or perforation of the oral mucosa occurs. These children should receive oral amoxicillin, and in allergic patients, clindamycin, 30–60 min before the intervention. No prophylaxis is recommended for other respiratory, gastrointestinal, or urinary procedures. The heart conditions for which this prophylaxis is indicated include cyanotic congenital heart disease, previous cardiac surgery with use of prosthetic material for repair of cardiac valve or congenital heart defects, and those with a previous history of IE. Parents and children with IE should maintain good oral hygiene. Infections with organisms likely to cause IE should be promptly treated with appropriate antibiotics.

11. *Should this Staphylococcus aureus IE detected in a child who developed a fever 1 week after discharge from the PICU be considered a hospital-acquired infection (HAI)?*

Yes. *Staphylococcus aureus* is a common cause of HAI and may become apparent 1 week after an ICU stay. Critically ill children in the PICU have a weakened immune system due to the severity of illness or immunosuppressive treatments. In the PICU, they are exposed to other patients with infections, health-care personnel, and possibly contaminated equipment or surfaces. Invasive procedures, such as central venous catheterization, ventilation, and urinary catheterization can introduce the organism into the bloodstream. Indwelling devices, such as central venous catheters, urinary catheters, and endotracheal tubes, increase the risk. Prolonged antibiotic use in the ICU can lead to the selection of antibiotic-resistant strains of *Staphylococcus aureus*, such as methicillin-resistant *Staphylococcus aureus* (MRSA). Even a short-term use of central venous catheters (CVCs) can pose a risk for IE as it provides a potential route for bacteria to enter the bloodstream. Also, the presence of a catheter within a blood vessel can disrupt the endothelial lining, making it easier for bacteria to adhere to the endothelium.

19.2 Conclusion

The child was continued on IV vancomycin. On day 4 of hospitalization, a soft grade 2 pansystolic murmur became detectable in the tricuspid area. The patient became afebrile on day 7. The antibiotics were continued for a total of 6 weeks. Repeat echocardiography showed a significant decrease in the size of vegetation. The patient was discharged in a stable condition with no fever and a weight gain of 2 kg.

Learning Points

1. Infective endocarditis is responsible for about 5% of cases of PUO in children.
2. Awareness among pediatricians is needed for prompt diagnosis.
3. Though congenital heart disease is the most common risk factor, over one-third (35.4%) of cases of IE in children occur in those without a pre-existing cardiac disease.
4. The symptoms of IE are nonspecific, and subtle, and in right-sided IE the murmur may not be audible.
5. In PUO with pulmonary infiltrates and anemia, TVIE should be suspected.
6. Blood cultures with optimal volume are absolutely essential in any PUO, and serial cultures are a must if IE is suspected.
7. Echocardiography should be done at the earliest in a child with PUO to identify IE.
8. Prompt initiation of appropriate antibiotics is needed to prevent complications and reduce mortality in IE.
9. The possibility of HAI should always be considered when fever develops in a child soon after discharge, especially after a stay in the PICU.
10. When there is persistent *Staphylococcus aureus* bacteremia even after initiation of appropriate antibiotics, metastatic infections including IE should be ruled out.
11. Even a short-term use of central venous catheters (CVCs) can pose a risk for IE as it provides a potential route for bacteria to enter the bloodstream.
12. Strict aseptic techniques during central line insertion and maintenance and prompt removal of the line when it is no longer necessary will minimize the risk of catheter-related infections including IE.

Suggested Readings

Lin YT, Hsieh KS, Chen YS, Huang IF, Cheng MF. Infective endocarditis in children without underlying heart disease. J Microbiol Immunol Infect. 2013;46(2):121–8. Epub 2012 Jun 23. https://doi.org/10.1016/j.jmii.2012.05.001.

Ranjan P, Kumar V, Ganguly S, Vyas S, Yadav R, Sood R. Isolated native tricuspid valve endocarditis presenting as PUO in a young adult male without any risk factors. J Fam Med Primary Care. 2015;4:139–41. Source of Support.

Shmueli H, Thomas F, Flint N, Setia G, Janjic A, Siegel RJ. Right-sided infective endocarditis 2020: challenges and updates in diagnosis and treatment. J Am Heart Assoc. 2020;9:e017293. https://doi.org/10.1161/JAHA.120.017293.

Vicent L, Luna R, Martínez-Sellés M. Pediatric infective endocarditis: a literature review. J Clin Med. 2022;11(11):3217. PMID: 35683606; PMCID: PMC9181776. https://doi.org/10.3390/jcm11113217.

Vasculitis

20

Contents

> **Key Messages**
> Inflammatory disorders like vasculitis can present as pyrexia of known origin (PUO). A careful examination of the peripheral pulses is an important component of the physical examination of children with PUO.

20.1 Case Discussion

A 17-year-old girl presented with low-grade intermittent fever for 1 month with a dull headache, reduced appetite, and weight loss. She was studying in class XI but attending school irregularly due to the headache. The headache had no specific character or aggravating/relieving factors. There were no visual symptoms or those of increased intracranial pressure (ICP). There were no other localizing symptoms involving the respiratory, gastrointestinal, musculoskeletal, or genitourinary systems, skin rashes, joint pains, or mucosal lesions. There was no contact history of tuberculosis. The child had received two courses of antibiotics and was on frequent doses of paracetamol for headache.

On examination, she was pale with a weight of 40 kg (below third centile), height of 152 cm (fifth centile), and body mass index (BMI) of 19.3 (between 25th and 50th centiles). She was afebrile, with a heart rate of 78/min and a respiratory rate of 28/min. Blood pressure in her left upper limb was documented as 100/60 mmHg. There were no palpable lymph nodes. Cardiac auscultation revealed S1 and S2 within normal limits. There were no murmurs, rubs, or gallops. Respiratory auscultation showed bilateral air entry and normal vesicular breath sounds, with no added sounds. The abdomen was soft to palpate, with no organomegaly. Neurologic examination including cranial nerves and spinal motor system, and ocular fundi were normal.

1. *What would be the differential diagnosis at this point?*

Given the history of prolonged fever with weight loss, without any localizing symptoms and no significant findings on examination and in

P. Venkat Ramanan, R. Padmanabhan, *Fever in Children*,
https://doi.org/10.1007/978-981-97-9967-1_20

view of the age and female sex, the possibility of a connective tissue disorder should be considered. Chronic infections like tuberculosis should also be ruled out. Investigations should be directed at confirming and/or ruling out the most likely diagnosis based on the history and examination.

With the clinical differentials listed above, she was investigated. Laboratory investigations revealed anemia (hemoglobin 10 g/dL) and elevated erythrocyte sedimentation rate (ESR, 71 mm/h). Peripheral smear and iron studies were suggestive of iron deficiency. Urine examination, total leucocyte count and platelet counts, and liver and kidney function tests were within normal limits. The Mantoux test was negative. Chest X-ray was normal. Rheumatoid factor, antinuclear factor, anti-double-stranded DNA antibodies, and antineutrophil cytoplasmic antibodies were negative. Complement factors C3 and C4 were normal.

2. *With the above investigations being normal, what would be the next step?*

In pyrexia of unknown origin (PUO), hospitalization for observation and frequent re-examination of the child are essential. Previously missed clinical signs can be picked up. Many diseases evolve slowly and new findings may appear. Frequent communication and frank discussion with the parents is essential as they will be quite anxious.

The child was re-examined and the blood pressure was recorded manually (previously recorded by the nurse using a noninvasive BP (NIBP) machine). In the right arm, it was noted to be 148/90 mmHg, more than the 95th percentile (95th percentile BP for age, gender, and height centile being 131/84 mmHg). The measurement of blood pressure manually on the left upper arm was difficult but was about 100/60 mmHg, as previously documented. The blood pressures on right and left lower limbs were 132/74 and 134/70 mmHg, respectively. On careful examination of her pulses, the left brachial and radial pulses were noted to be significantly weaker than the right. Auscultation over the major vessels revealed no bruit. Re-examination of central nervous system, and fundoscopic eye examination was normal.

In view of the hypertension noted in the right upper limb, the difference in the four-limb blood pressures, and the difficulty in palpating the left radial and brachial pulses, a clinical diagnosis of Takayasu arteritis (TAK) was made.

3. *Is it necessary to measure the blood pressure manually with all the advances in automated technology currently available?*

There are advantages and disadvantages to both methods. The manual method requires training and takes a little more time. Hence, electronic devices have become popular. In many clinics nowadays, once the patient is registered, the pulse rate and SpO_2 are noted by the nurse using the pulse oximeter and the arterial blood pressure is measured using the non-invasive BP (NIBP) machine. So palpation of the pulses is overlooked. A careful examination of all the peripheral pulses in an important component of the physical examination of children, more so in a child with PUO. The manual method of recording the blood pressure is especially important for patients with hypertension, hypotension, or pulse irregularities.

4. *What is Takayasu arteritis and what are the clinical features?*

Takayasu arteritis (TAK) is an inflammatory condition of the vessel wall mainly involving the aorta and its branches, the subclavian and carotid arteries. The etiology is unknown. It primarily affects women, and the usual age of onset is between 10 and 40 years. As the inflammation progresses, stenoses form and collaterals may develop.

The clinical features range from asymptomatic disease recognized incidentally by impalpable pulse or bruits to serious organ impairment due to ischemia caused by stenosis. The common early clinical features are nonspecific and include constitutional symptoms like weakness, malaise, fever, weight loss, arthralgia, myalgia, and mild anemia. As the inflammation continues, progressive narrowing, occlusion, or dilation of arteries occurs. Diminished or absent pulses can be seen in 84% to 96% of TAK patients; vascular bruits in 80% to 94%; hypertension in 33% to 83%; and retinopathy is seen in 37% of patients. Hypertension is due to narrowing of one or both renal arteries, or narrowing and decreased elasticity of the aorta and branches. Falsely low blood pressure in one or both arms is common due to narrowing or occlusion of the arteries in the arms; a difference of more than 10 mmHg between the arms is typical. Sometimes, it is difficult to assess the blood pressure in the upper limbs, and BP has to be measured using an appropriate size in an uninvolved lower limb. Symptoms related to organs that receive blood from the vessels affected include pain in the hand or lower leg with use (claudication), abdominal pain especially after eating, angina, respiratory symptoms, and neurological symptoms.

5. *What are the investigations that help in diagnosing TAK?*

Early diagnosis and institution of treatment can prevent damage accrual. Erythrocyte sedimentation rate (ESR) and highly sensitive serum C-reactive protein (hsCRP) levels are usually elevated and are used to monitor disease activity and guide therapy. They are nonspecific, and research is ongoing to identify novel biomarkers. A clinical diagnosis of TAK can be made in a patient when there are suggestive clinical features with hypertension, diminished or absent pulses, and/or arterial bruits, and imaging showing narrowing of the aorta and/or its primary branches.

When vasculitis is suspected, vascular imaging should be done and angiography is the gold standard for visualizing arterial involvement and assessing the extent of the disease. It helps in identifying stenotic lesions, aneurysms, and vascular occlusions. Commonly, imaging methods such as Doppler ultrasound, computed tomography (CT) angiography, or magnetic resonance angiography (MRA) are used (Fig. 20.1). These, in addition to visualizing the arterial lumen, provide valuable information about inflammation in the arterial wall and periarterial structures, thus

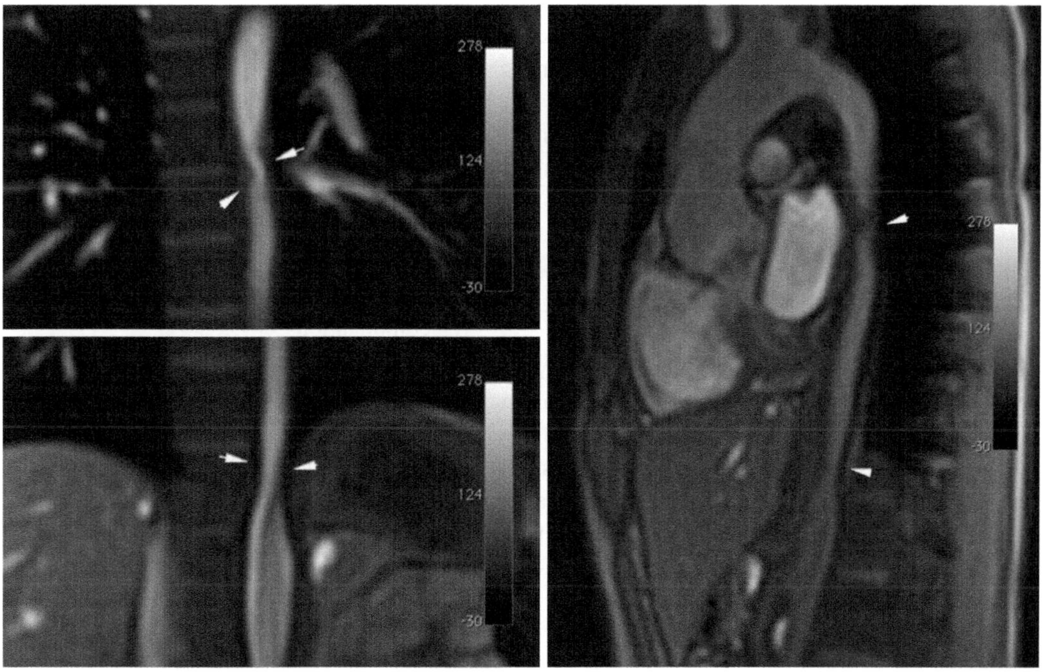

Fig. 20.1 MRA showing narrowing of the descending aorta at two locations with the evidence of inflammation and edema of the aortic wall. (Photo courtesy Dr. Jebaraj R)

facilitating the diagnosis at an early stage, in which arterial wall thickening is present and the lumen diameter is preserved. The use of positron emission tomography utilizing 18F-FDG (FDG PET scan) often in combination with CT (PET-CT) in the workup of PUO has improved case detection rates. The finding of "hot" segments in large vessels may suggest large-vessel vasculitis, and it can also measure the intensity of the vessel wall involvement.

In this child, MRA was done which revealed aortic arch vessel involvement with narrowing at the left subclavian artery and in the descending aorta (Fig. 20.1). The diagnosis of Takayasu arteritis was confirmed.

6. *What is the treatment of TAK?*

TAK is a chronic inflammatory disease with remissions and exacerbations of the inflammatory process. Active TAK is treated initially with high-dose, oral glucocorticoids along with a glucocorticoid-sparing agent like methotrexate or azathioprine. Antihypertensives are needed to control the high blood pressure, and ACE inhibitors should be avoided until renal artery stenosis has been excluded. Low- dose aspirin is used empirically, especially, when there is critical stenosis of more than one artery. Stenosed or occluded arteries leading to organ ischemia and aneurysm need surgical management.

20.2 Conclusion

She was referred to the Pediatric Rheumatology services where she was treated initially with oral prednisolone 1 mg/kg/day and weekly oral methotrexate, aspirin, and antihypertensives. She responded well and became afebrile within a week. The oral steroids were tapered off after 4 weeks. The patient is currently on methotrexate, aspirin, and antihypertensives, and on regular follow-up, she continues to be in remission.

Learning Points

1. Although infections are standard differentials for PUO in the low and middle-income countries (LMIC), inflammatory disorders like vasculitis should also be considered.
2. Takayasu arteritis (TAK) (pulseless disease) may present as PUO; in the pre-pulseless phase, the symptoms are nonspecific.
3. Careful palpation of all peripheral pulses and blood pressure recording are essential in evaluating any child with PUO. Tenderness along arteries, bruits, and aneurysm may point to the diagnosis.
4. TAK, a large-vessel vasculitis of unknown etiology, predominantly affects young females, and it has an early inflammatory phase and a late chronic phase.
5. The early inflammatory phase, lasting for weeks to months, is characterized by nonspecific symptoms such as fever, malaise, night sweats, loss of appetite, and weight loss, but TAK is rarely diagnosed in this phase.
6. Symptoms in the chronic phase are due to arterial stenosis/occlusion and ischemia of organs. Clinical manifestations are related to the location of arterial lesions.
7. Early diagnosis and treatment of TAK are essential to prevent vascular complications.
8. Treatment involves immunosuppressants such as prednisone and/or methotrexate to decrease or eliminate inflammatory activity.
9. Hypertension should be treated aggressively, often with a multidrug regimen.
10. ACE inhibitors should be avoided until renal artery stenosis has been excluded.

Acknowledgments We thank Dr. Jebaraj, Pediatric cardiologist, and Dr. Mahesh Janardhanan, Pediatric rheumatologist at Sri Ramachandra Hospital, for their valuable input in managing the case and retrieving the MRA images from their archives.

Suggested Readings

Aeschlimann FA, Yeung RSM, Laxer RM. An update on childhood-onset Takayasu arteritis. Front Pediatr. 2022;10:872313. https://doi.org/10.3389/fped.2022.872313.

Brunner J, Feldman BM, Tyrrell PN, et al. Takayasu arteritis in children and adolescents. Rheumatology (Oxford). 2010;49:1806.

European League Against Rheumatism (EULAR). Recommendations for the management of large vessel vasculitis. 2018 update (published 2019).

Part III

Recurrent Fever

21 Factitious Fever

Contents

Key Messages
In a child with a history of recurrent, high-grade fever, who is otherwise healthy-looking, the possibility of factitious fever should be considered when all reports are normal. The clinical clues include a persistently normal temperature when not self-measured, the absence of tachycardia, and malaise or discomfort during fever, and a rapid defervescence of the fever without diaphoresis.

21.1 Case Discussion

A 14-year-old boy, studying in Class 9 in a residential school, was brought to the outpatient department with a history of recurrent episodes of fever for 3 months. This time, he had a history of fever for 3 days. The child had been admitted into the residential school last June, and the episodes had started within a month of joining. The fever episodes usually started abruptly with a maximum recorded temperature of 104.4 °F and lasted for 1 to 2 days. He was having two to three such episodes every month. They were sometimes associated with headache but no respiratory, urinary, or gastrointestinal symptoms. The school doctors had not found any focus of infection. The boy shared a room with three other students, and viral respiratory infections were common among the students in the dorm. He had been investigated in the school clinic previously for common febrile illnesses and the reports were found to be normal. The episodes had been treated symptomatically as viral fever. As the episodes became frequent, his parents were asked to take him home and have him evaluated. There was no history of tiredness or weight loss. In fact, he had gained 2 kg after joining the residential school.

He had taken all his childhood vaccines and had no significant past history. His parents were both hospital staff, and his younger sister was in Class 5. He had scored 62% marks in his eighth standard exams, and his parents had admitted him to the residential school for better supervision of his studies. The boy said he had no major problems at school but the fever episodes caused

P. Venkat Ramanan, R. Padmanabhan, *Fever in Children*,
https://doi.org/10.1007/978-981-97-9967-1_21

him to miss classes. On examination, he was overweight, alert, and had normal vital signs. The axillary temperature measured in the outpatient department was 98.2 °F. General physical examination and systemic examination were normal.

1. *What is "recurrent fever" and what are the causes of recurrent fever in children?*

The term "recurrent fever" in adults refers to ≥3 fever episodes in a 6-month period, occurring at least 7 days apart, with no causative medical illness. These episodes may occur at regular or irregular intervals. There is no widely accepted definition for children. Recurrent respiratory infections are a common cause of recurrent fevers in young children, and most of these episodes are due to self-limiting viral infections. However, they are less common in adolescence. The differential diagnosis is long and has been discussed in detail in Chap. 23.

2. *What are the investigations recommended in this boy at this stage?*

Diagnostic testing should be guided by history and focused physical examination. When physical examination is normal, the initial investigations would be a complete blood count, urine routine examination, blood and urine cultures, erythrocyte sedimentation rate, and a chest X-ray for tuberculosis.

The child was investigated. His hemoglobin level was 14.2 g/dL, total leucocyte count was 5200 cells/cmm, differential count and platelet counts were normal, and ESR was 7 mm first hour. The chest X-ray and urine routine reports were also normal. Blood and urine cultures were normal.

3. *How should we proceed?*

Since these reports are normal, a "wait and watch" approach with careful follow-up alone is recommended. The disease has to evolve before some clue to the underlying cause emerges. Before any test is ordered, there should be a well-considered differential diagnosis. For example, when there is no lymphadenopathy or organomegaly and the complete blood count and peripheral smears are normal, a positive bone marrow tap is unlikely. With a normal ESR, autoimmune disorders and malignancy are unlikely.

The parents were asked to maintain a temperature record at home and return when the fever recurred. Six days later, the boy was brought back to the emergency room at 7.15 a.m. with a reported fever of 105.4 °F since 6 a.m. He had been afebrile for the last 5 days, and the parents planned to take him back to school that morning. In the ER, the temperature documented by the nurse was normal. There was no history of intake of any antipyretic drugs and no sweating. On examination, he was cool to touch, his vital signs were normal, his physical examination was normal, and he seemed comfortable. As the boy was otherwise comfortable and cheerful, he was asked to continue maintaining a temperature record at home and return after 48 h. He returned after 48 h with a temperature record showing fever spikes of 103 to 105 °F every 4 h. There were no associated symptoms, and the temperature recorded by the clinic nurse was normal. This time, the boy said he had taken paracetamol before coming to the hospital but no diaphoresis was noted. In view of the previously normal reports, the dramatic drop in his body temperature within an hour with no sweating, and the overall demeanor of the child, the possibility of factitious fever was considered.

4. *What is factitious fever?*

Factitious fever is a false report of fever given by a caregiver or patient, or fabricating a false thermometer reading by dipping the thermometer bulb into something hot, by manipulation of body temperature by rinsing the mouth with hot water or keeping a hot-water bag under the axilla. Rarely, fevers are actually induced by the injection of infective or foreign materials, by an older patient or by a parent/caregiver. Around 9% of cases of fevers of unknown origin or recurrent infections were factitious or self-induced, but the possibility should be considered only after exclusion of organic illness.

Factitious fever can result in overuse of healthcare services as well as harm to these patients because of unnecessary medication, repeated investigations, and invasive examinations.

On further questioning, the mother said the boy had always been recording his own body temperature with a digital thermometer in the axilla and showing the value to the mother once it started beeping. She said she had never actually recorded the temperature herself during the episodes or felt him to see if he was hot. The child was hospitalized for observation.

5. *When should factitious fever be suspected?*

Factitious fever should be suspected when there is a history of persistent/recurrent fever without weight loss, with incongruities in medical history, clinical examination, and laboratory findings. The clues to a factitious fever include a normal temperature when not self-measured, absence of tachycardia, and malaise or discomfort in a patient with high fever, rapid defervescence without diaphoresis, and extreme hyperpyrexia. The body temperature is usually recorded in the axilla and sometimes oral cavity. The temperature of freshly voided urine, collected in a plastic cup and measured immediately after voiding reflects the core body temperature. It is one way to verify if only the surface body temperature has been recorded.

After hospitalization, the child was asked to continue recording his own body temperature like he used to do at home and in his boarding school and note it down. While he was showing thermometer recordings to be between 101 °F and 104 °F, the temperature recorded by the nurses was always found to be normal. During his stay, the nurses also noticed that he always spent sometime in the bathroom before coming out and recording his axillary temperature. He was subsequently noted to often have hot towels under his arms beneath his shirt which he said was to help control shivering.

6. *When feigned illness is suspected what is the subsequent management?*

The suspicion should be discussed within the team of health-care providers, and all members of the team should behave with an attitude of professionalism and empathy. When there are sufficient indicators, the patient and his parents should be informed about the differential diagnosis and confronted in a stepwise, supportive manner. It should be explained that the patient's psychological distress is the cause of fever, and full assurance should be given that they will continue to receive active care. They should be offered the opportunities of psychotherapy, and the underlying psychological factors driving the behavior should be addressed. Some patients may take this offer, while others may deny feigning illness to avoid loss of face and embarrassment, but stop feigning after a confrontation. A hostile approach will make these patients switch doctors and continuing their deception in other institutions.

21.2 Conclusion

A family meeting was held during which the observations made in the hospital were shared. Once confronted, the family shared long-held suspicions that he was manipulating his body temperature. The parents were counseled to avoid harsh or sarcastic comments and a psychiatrist consultation was recommended. The patient revealed feeling homesick in his residential school but also feeling unloved and neglected at home. He felt his parents were busy with their careers and that they loved his sister more as she was scoring better marks at school. He was discharged with referrals for outpatient mental health follow-up and family counseling.

Learning Points

1. Around 9% of cases of fevers of unknown origin or recurrent infections were factitious or self-induced.
2. The possibility of factitious fever should be considered only after exclusion of organic illness.

3. The clues to a factitious fever include incongruities in medical history, a normal temperature when not self-measured, absence of tachycardia, and malaise or discomfort in a patient with high fever, rapid defervescence without diaphoresis, and extreme hyperpyrexia.
4. Tests should not be needlessly repeated without a clinical indication in the hope that a pathology will be suddenly found.
5. When suspected, the patient and the parents should be informed about the differential diagnosis and confronted in a stepwise, supportive manner with professionalism and empathy.
6. Family counseling and psychotherapy should be offered and harsh or sarcastic comments should be avoided.

Suggested Readings

Feldman MD, Yates GP. Dying to be ill: true stories of medical deception. New York: Routledge; 2018.

Hausteiner-Wiehle C, Hungerer S. Factitious disorders in everyday clinical practice. Dtsch Arztebl Int. 2020;117(26):452–9. PMID: 32897184; PMCID: PMC7505250. https://doi.org/10.3238/arztebl.2020.0452.

Tatu L, Aybek S, Bogousslavsky J. Munchausen syndrome and the wide spectrum of factitious disorders. Front Neurol Neurosci. 2018;42:81–6.

Sarcoidosis

22

Contents

> **Key Messages**
> Pediatric sarcoidosis is a multisystem disorder that may present with nonspecific systemic symptoms, such as fever, fatigue, and weight loss, as well as symptoms related to the involved organs: the lungs, eyes, skin, and lymph nodes. Careful examination of the skin for rashes/nodules and the eyes for uveitis, even when there are no eye symptoms, is important in evaluating children with recurrent fever.

22.1 Case Discussion

A 4-year-old boy presented with a history of recurrent fever for 4 months, each episode lasting for 2–3 weeks, interspersed with afebrile period of 4–6 weeks. The episodes were associated with reduced appetite, easy fatiguability, and occasional joint pains but no obvious joint swelling or tenderness. There were no other localizing symptoms. The child was not going to daycare or a regular school. He had not gained or lost weight in the previous 4 months. He was the only child of a non-consanguineous marriage without a significant family history. There was no history of contact with animals. On examination, his weight and height were on the third percentile for age. He was afebrile and alert. He had mild pallor, and the general physical examination was otherwise normal. His systemic examination, including musculoskeletal system examination, was also normal.

1. *What would be the differential diagnosis in a child with recurrent fever?*

Recurrent fever can be due to infectious or noninfectious causes. The most common cause in young children is recurrent episodes of independent uncomplicated viral upper respiratory tract infections, especially in children who begin going to school or daycare. Subacute infections such as tuberculosis, brucellosis, infective endocarditis, melioidosis, and occult abscesses are typically characterized by prolonged fever rather than recurrent fever. Other infections to be

P. Venkat Ramanan, R. Padmanabhan, *Fever in Children*,
https://doi.org/10.1007/978-981-97-9967-1_22

considered in India include malaria and visceral leishmaniasis. The noninfectious causes of recurrent fever are autoimmune and granulomatous diseases, periodic fever syndromes, autoinflammatory disorders, underlying immunodeficiency, and malignancies.

A good clinical history, physical examination findings, and targeted investigations can help narrow the differential diagnosis.

In this child, in view of the long duration of the illness, malignancy was considered less likely and the child was investigated. A complete blood count revealed a hemoglobin level of 9.2 g/dL with normal total and differential leucocyte counts. The C-reactive protein (CRP) was 0.6 mg/dL (ref. range < 0.6), and the erythrocyte sedimentation rate was 46 mm in the first hour (normal <20). Peripheral blood smear showed no atypical cells or hemoparasites. Urine analysis was normal. Liver and kidney function tests were normal. The chest radiography and abdominal ultrasound were normal. The tuberculin skin test was negative.

As the ESR was elevated, with almost all infective workup being negative, the possibility of a connective tissue disease was considered. Serological evaluations for autoantibodies (antinuclear antibody, anti-ds-DNA) were negative.

During the hospital stay, the child was noted to rub his eyes frequently. The mother said he had been complaining of irritation for several weeks and was sensitive to bright lights. She had attributed these symptoms to excessive TV watching. The child was sent for a complete ophthalmology evaluation. A slit lamp ophthalmic examination revealed anterior uveitis (Fig. 22.1).

2. *When should uveitis be suspected in children?*

Pediatricians need to specifically inquire about symptoms of uveitis in children with unexplained fever and those at risk due to their rheumatological conditions. The clinical features depend on the extent, location, and severity of ocular inflammation and range from asymptomatic to eye pain, irritation, and visual symptoms. The diagnosis of uveitis is challenging for several reasons. The onset is insidious; young children do not consistently report their symptoms, and eye examination for young children is difficult and needs experience.

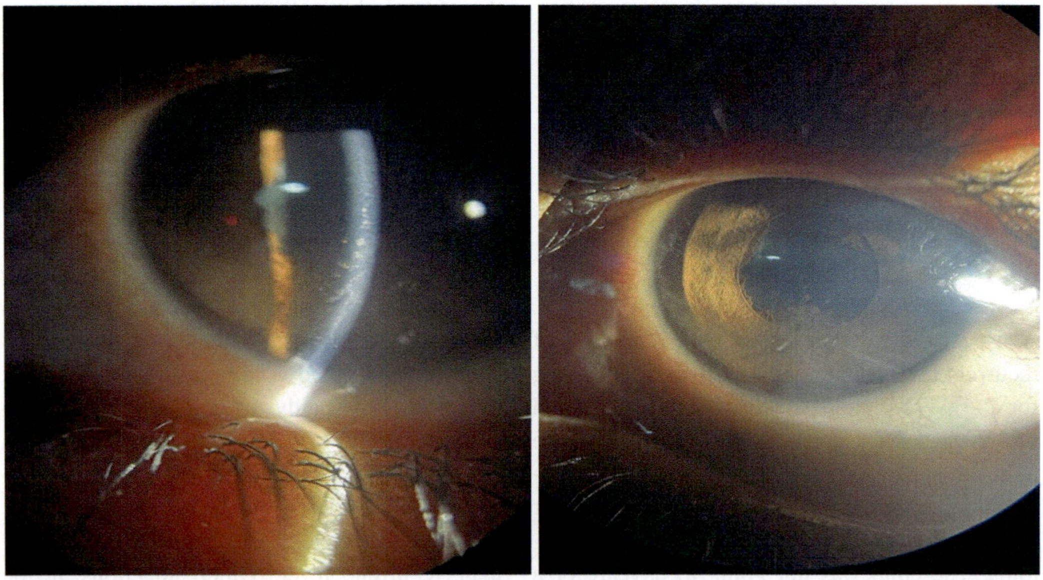

Fig. 22.1 Slit lamp examination showing active anterior uveitis (left) and resolving uveitis (right). (Photos courtesy Dr. Radha Annamalai)

3. *What are the conditions that can cause recurrent fever and uveitis in children?*

Uveitis is seen in infections such as tuberculosis, syphilis, toxoplasmosis, histoplasmosis, Lyme disease, and several viral infections. Noninfectious uveitis is seen in juvenile idiopathic arthritis, inflammatory bowel disease, SLE, sarcoidosis, and some forms of vasculitis. In a child with uveitis, history is the key to recognizing symptoms of extraocular involvement, which gives a clue to the underlying cause. It's important to look for rashes, joint pain, cough, shortness of breath, bowel symptoms, and hearing loss.

4. *With this differential diagnosis, what should be the next step?*

Repeat clinical examination revealed two well-defined, slightly raised firm plaques on both the shins (1.2 cm × 1.1 cm and 1.4 cm × 1 cm), and the lesion was biopsied. Hematoxylin and eosin-stained sections from the lesion revealed naked epithelioid cell granulomas (granulomas without significant surrounding lymphoid infiltrate) in the deep dermis with minimal areas of necrosis (Fig. 22.2).

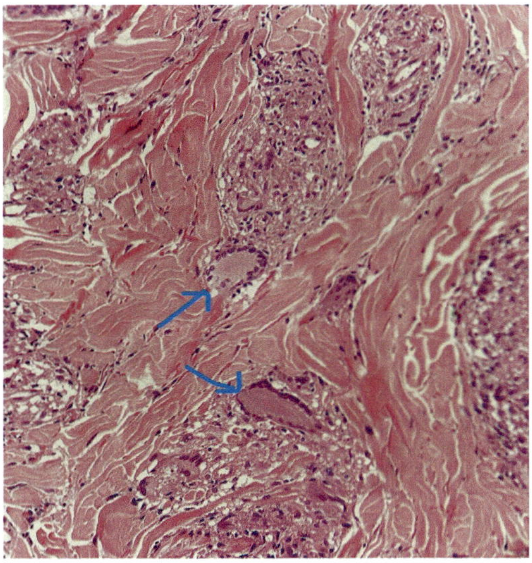

Fig. 22.2 Photomicrograph showing granulomas with giant cells (arrows) H&E × 200. (Photos courtesy Dr. Leena Dennis Joseph)

The possibility of sarcoidosis was considered. Serum and urine calcium levels were normal, but serum angiotensin-converting enzyme (ACE) level was raised (78 U/L; normal range 8–65 U/L). Since all other infective workup was negative, a diagnosis of sarcoidosis was made. The child was treated with corticosteroids and methotrexate.

5. *What is sarcoidosis, and how does it present in children?*

Sarcoidosis is a multisystem granulomatous disorder that affects mainly young or middle-aged adults. It is uncommon in children, and the incidence of clinically recognized sarcoidosis in children is estimated to be 0.22 to 0.29/100,000 children per year. Non-necrotizing inflammatory granulomas and subsequent fibrosis in the lungs and other organs cause the symptoms. Clinical manifestations vary widely, depending on the organ involved.

Childhood sarcoidosis presents in two distinct patterns-one in children younger than 5 years of age and the other in older children. Children < 5 years of age tend to have skin, ophthalmic, and joint disease without significant pulmonary involvement (Blau syndrome). Blau syndrome (BS) and early-onset sarcoidosis (EOS) have been identified as familial and sporadic phenotypes of the same non-caseating granulomatous form caused by CARD15/NOD2 gene mutations.

Older children (age 8–15 years) have a disease pattern like adults with systemic symptoms and multisystem involvement of lungs, lymph nodes, eyes, bones, and skin. Systemic manifestations include fever, fatigue, generalized lymphadenopathy, and weight loss. Lung involvement may cause cough, dyspnea, fatigue, and chest pain. The prognosis and natural history of childhood sarcoidosis are not clearly described due to the rarity of the disease and the paucity of literature.

6. *What are the ocular and cutaneous features of sarcoidosis?*

Sarcoidosis can affect any part of the eye. It may cause anterior, intermediate, posterior, or pan uveitis. The other ocular manifestations include dry eye due to lacrimal gland involvement, scleritis, and optic neuritis. Conjunctival or choroidal granulomas and peripheral multifocal choroiditis are considered specific markers of ocular sarcoidosis; however, it is anterior uveitis or iritis that occurs more frequently and leads to considerable morbidity.

Cutaneous sarcoidosis may present in several forms: papular, plaque, nodular, macular, and rarely ichthyosiform or psoriasiform. Nonspecific lesions such as erythema nodosum or pyoderma gangrenosum may occur alone or coexist with specific sarcoidosis lesions.

7. *What is the etiopathogenesis of sarcoidosis?*

In sarcoidosis, there is chronic inflammation and granuloma formation in the target organs. These granulomas mediate disease by secreting cytokines that provoke constitutional symptoms and triggering inflammation that may cause irreversible organ damage. These granulomas either resolve or heal by fibrosis. The cause of sarcoidosis is not known. It is believed to occur when a genetically susceptible host is exposed to an environmental trigger that causes an exaggerated immune response, leading to granuloma formation. The trigger could be an infectious agent.

8. *What are the tests required to confirm the diagnosis of sarcoidosis?*

There is no single diagnostic test for sarcoidosis. The diagnosis is made with specific pathologic and radiographic features in appropriate clinical settings. Chest radiographs (X-ray/CT scan) must be done in all cases. Bilateral hilar lymphadenopathy is seen in 50% of cases. Lung parenchyma may show nodular, reticular, or ground-glass opacities that may be generalized or localized to the mid or upper lung zones. HRCT of the chest can detect smaller lesions often missed in chest X-ray. The characteristic feature of sarcoidosis is small nodules (2 to 5 mm) in a perilymphatic distribution in the lung parenchyma and bilateral, symmetrical hilar involvement. Ophthalmic slit lamp examination for typical findings of sarcoidosis should be done in all patients. Elevated serum ACE levels and ESR are useful indicators of disease activity. A biopsy is done from the most accessible site, and the histopathologic finding is non-necrotizing granulomas in the involved organ systems. Enlarged peripheral lymph nodes seen in nearly 70% of patients are the most accessible tissue for biopsy. It is important to rule out granulomatous infection, especially tuberculosis and histoplasmosis.

9. *What is the sensitivity and specificity of ACE level in diagnosing sarcoidosis? In which other conditions can it be raised?*

Angiotensin-converting enzyme (ACE) is produced by the activated macrophages that form the epithelioid cells of the granuloma. Hence, its serum level increases with the number of granulomas in the body and disease severity. Serum ACE level is also elevated in other granulomatous diseases, such as tuberculosis, leprosy, and histoplasmosis, and in some non-granulomatous diseases, such as hyperthyroidism, Gaucher disease, and Hodgkin lymphoma. The sensitivity of elevated serum ACE level for diagnosis of sarcoidosis is approximately 42%. When ACE level is raised to more than twice the upper limit of normal, the specificity is 90%.

10. *How is sarcoidosis treated?*

Treatment of sarcoidosis focuses on reducing and preventing inflammation and granuloma formation that cause organ dysfunction due to fibrosis. The disease clears spontaneously in approximately 50% of patients. Glucocorticoids are the drug of choice for children with multisystem involvement. Low-dose oral methotrexate (MTX) is safe and effective and has a steroid-sparing effect. There is limited experience with other immunosuppressive agents used in adult sarcoidosis such as azathioprine, cyclophosphamide, chlorambucil, and cyclosporine.

22.2 Conclusion

The child became afebrile on corticosteroids and methotrexate, and the ACE levels and ESR normalized in 6 weeks. The parents were counseled regarding the need for genetic studies.

Learning Points

1. Sarcoidosis, a multisystem granulomatous disorder, is a rare cause of recurrent fever in children.
2. The most common manifestations of sarcoidosis in children over 5 years of age are systemic symptoms (fever, fatigue, generalized lymphadenopathy) followed by symptoms of eye involvement.
3. Complete ophthalmic evaluation and careful skin examination for rashes and/or nodules are important components of the evaluation of a child with recurrent or prolonged fever.
4. Childhood sarcoidosis should be considered among the differential diagnosis of uveitis and atypical cutaneous lesions.
5. In children below 5, sarcoidosis typically presents with skin, ophthalmic, and joint disease, with or without fever, associated with CARD15/NOD2 gene mutations.
6. There is no single diagnostic test for sarcoidosis; the diagnosis rests primarily on demonstrating non-caseating epithelioid granulomas on histopathological examination of biopsy from the affected organs.
7. Enlarged peripheral lymph nodes seen in nearly 70% of patients are the most accessible tissue for biopsy.
8. Other causes of granulomatous disease have to be excluded, especially mycobacterial and fungal infections.
9. Serum ACE levels are elevated in 40–75% of patients with sarcoidosis.
10. The treatment of pediatric sarcoidosis is with corticosteroids and low-dose methotrexate.

Suggested Readings

Chiu B, Chan J, Das S, Alshamma Z, Sergi C. Pediatric sarcoidosis: a review with emphasis on early onset and high-risk sarcoidosis and diagnostic challenges. Diagnostics (Basel). 2019;9(4):160. PMID: 31731423; PMCID: PMC6963233. https://doi.org/10.3390/diagnostics9040160.

Gedalia A, Khan TA, Shetty AK, Dimitriades VR, Espinoza LR. Childhood sarcoidosis: Louisiana experience. Clin Rheumatol. 2016;35(7):1879–84. Epub 2015 Jan 24. https://doi.org/10.1007/s10067-015-2870-9.

Sangwan A, Kaur S, Aggarwal K, Dua I. Childhood sarcoidosis: an atypical case report. Indian J Dermatol. 2017;62(5):548. PMID: 28979033; PMCID: PMC5618858. https://doi.org/10.4103/ijd.IJD_658_16.

PFAPA (Periodic Fever, Aphthous Stomatitis, Pharyngitis, Cervical Adenitis) Syndrome

23

Contents

> **Key Messages**
> PFAPA (periodic fever, aphthous stomatitis, pharyngitis, cervical adenitis) syndrome is a common, but underdiagnosed cause of recurrent fever in young children. Aphthous ulcers are usually on the inner lips or buccal mucosa, and careful physical examination during flares is required to identify ulcers.

23.1 Case Discussion

A 4-year-old girl presented with a history of recurrent fevers for 1 year. The current episode of fever had begun 2 days ago. The febrile episodes were usually sudden in onset, associated with a temperature of 102–103 °F, and typically lasted for 3–5 days. There was a history of sore throat during some of the episodes during which the child was being treated with oral antibiotics. There was no history of rashes, joint pain, or swelling. She was otherwise active in the intervals between episodes, gaining weight and doing well in school. She had an elder brother aged 9 years who was normal. She had no significant medical history till the age of 3 years. She had received all her immunizations according to the national immunization schedule without any adverse reactions. There was no history of previous hospitalization or life -threatening infections. The parents reported that the doctors they had consulted in the past had always found her physical examination to be normal except for throat congestion. Her repeated blood and urine investigations also apparently had been noncontributory. As these episodes were occurring almost every month, the parents wanted to rule out major underlying illnesses.

On physical examination, her axillary temperature was 103.2 °F and other vital signs were normal. She was well grown and her general condition was good. Throat examination revealed hyperemic, congested pharynx and tonsils (Fig. 23.1).

P. Venkat Ramanan, R. Padmanabhan, *Fever in Children*,
https://doi.org/10.1007/978-981-97-9967-1_23

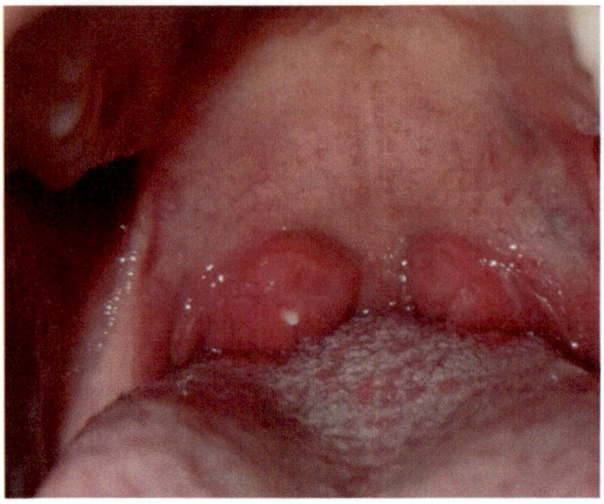

Fig. 23.1 Throat examination showing hyperemic tonsils. (Photo courtesy Dr. S. Prasanna Kumar)

1. *What are the causes of pharyngotonsillitis in children?*

Pharyngotonsillitis is usually due to a viral or bacterial infection. The common viruses that cause tonsillitis include rhinovirus, respiratory syncytial virus, adenovirus, and coronavirus. Other viruses like Epstein–Barr virus (EBV) (causing mononucleosis), cytomegalovirus, hepatitis A, rubella, and HIV may also cause tonsillitis. Bacterial tonsillitis is usually due to group A beta-hemolytic *Streptococcus* (GABHS) and can be diagnosed by throat culture or a rapid antigen detection test.

A clinical diagnosis of recurrent tonsillitis was made. Throat and blood cultures were sent and oral amoxicillin was started. She was also investigated for other possible causes of recurrent fever.

2. *What is the differential diagnosis of recurrent fevers in children?*

Recurrent fevers may be due to infectious or noninfectious causes.

(a) Infectious causes: The differential diagnosis of recurrent infections would depend upon the age and the severity of the infections. Recurrent episodes of minor self-limiting viral infections are usually due to environmental factors (smoking, daycare). Recurrent urinary tract infection (UTI) is also common in children. Recurrent episodes of serious viral, bacterial, or fungal infections suggest an underlying immunodeficiency when they affect multiple organs. When the infections are limited to a single organ system, the target system has to be evaluated for a predisposing cause.
(b) Autoimmune conditions and malignancies can cause recurring fevers and should be suspected when there is growth failure and persistence of other symptoms in between the fever episodes.
(c) Periodic fevers: When there is recurrent fever without an identifiable infection, the episodes are stereotypical, and the child is well in between the episodes, monogenic fever syndromes like familial Mediterranean fever (FMF) and hyper-Ig D syndrome, cyclical neutropenia (caused by gene mutation), and periodic fever, aphthous stomatitis, pharyngitis, and adenitis (PFAPA) syndrome (an auto-inflammatory condition) should be considered.
(d) Miscellaneous causes: Recurrent fever in infants, in the absence of sweating, should raise concern for diabetes insipidus, familial dysautonomia, or hypohidrotic ectodermal dysplasia. Recurrent episodes of fever associated with arm and leg pain may indicate Fabry disease.

Her blood tests showed leukocytosis (TLC 15,680/cmm) with a shift to the left, C-reactive protein value of 8 mg/dL, and erythrocyte sedimentation rate (ESR) of 24 mm/h. The blood and throat cultures were negative, and serological studies for Epstein–Barr virus (EBV) were also negative. The peripheral blood smear revealed normal findings. She had normal levels of C3 and C4 and serum immunoglobulin (Ig). Rheumatological tests including the antinuclear antibodies (ANA), anti-DNA antibodies, and rheumatoid factor were negative. Chest X-ray and abdominal ultrasonography showed normal findings.

On review on after 48 h, fever was persisting and the mother also complained that the child was refusing to eat even mildly spicy food. A

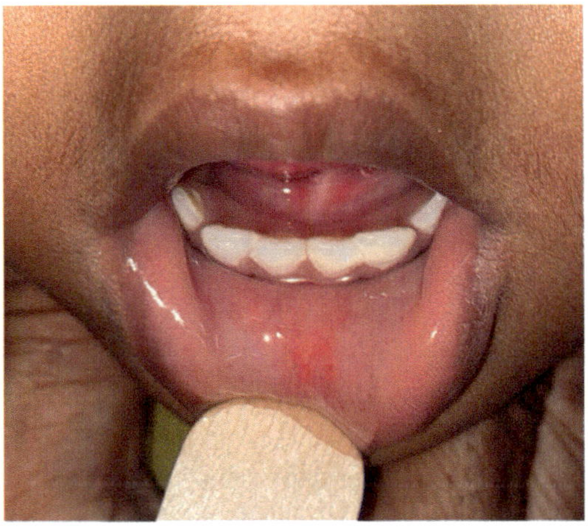

Fig. 23.2 Ulcers on the inner side of the lower lip. (Photo courtesy Dr. Dhanaratnamoorthy)

thorough physical examination was performed again. Repeat oral examination revealed small ulcers in the mucus membrane of the mouth (Fig. 23.2).

Based on these clinical features and the exclusion of other causes of recurrent fever, the possibility of periodic fever, aphthous stomatitis, pharyngitis, and adenitis (PFAPA) syndrome was considered. All antibiotics were stopped, and oral prednisolone was started.

3. *What is periodic fever, aphthous stomatitis, pharyngitis, and adenitis (PFAPA) syndrome?*

Periodic fever, aphthous stomatitis, pharyngitis, and adenitis (PFAPA) syndrome is the most common non genetic cause of recurrent fever in children. It is an auto-inflammatory disease which was first described by Marshall et al. in 1987, and in 1989, the acronym PFAPA was coined. The symptoms usually begin before the age of 5 years. There are episodes of high fever (>39 °C) that recur every 3 to 6 weeks. The fever is associated with pharyngitis and stomatitis in 67% of cases, and cervical reactive adenopathy in 77% of cases. Other minor symptoms include headache, abdominal pain, nausea, vomiting, chills, and malaise. These children are not immunodeficient. The episodes last for 4–6 days after which the symptoms resolve regardless of the antibiotic or antipyretic treatment. In between the episodes, these children remain asymptomatic and have a normal growth and development. The syndrome lasts for 4–5 years, with a progressive decrease of frequency and intensity.

4. *What is the cause of PFAPA?*

The etiology is still not well understood. It is an auto-inflammatory condition, and increased levels of inflammatory cytokines have been demonstrated during the fever episodes. It is believed that the tonsillar inflammation, lymphadenitis, and aphthous ulcers are immunologically mediated. It is different from autoimmune disorders in which there are autoantibodies or autoreactive T cells.

5. *What investigations help in the diagnosis?*

The diagnosis of this syndrome is clinical, and there are no diagnostic investigations. Blood investigations may show nonspecific leukocytosis and a moderate increase in the erythrocyte sedimentation rate (ESR) during the episodes. Investigations help in ruling out other causes of recurrent fever.

6. *If there are no diagnostic tests, how can we differentiate PFAPA syndrome from other causes of recurrent fever?*

A good history is important. The age of onset (1–4 years), the periodicity of the fever (every 2–8 weeks), the associated symptoms, and the abrupt resolution of symptoms without antibiotics or analgesics suggest PFAPA syndrome. The caregiver should be asked to note the dates of fever episodes and associated symptoms, and the pattern has to be analyzed carefully. The good general condition of the patient in between the episodes and normal growth are also pointers to the diagnosis. The dramatic response to a single dose of oral prednisolone supports the diagnosis and has been suggested as a diagnostic criterion.

Other causes of recurrent fever in children should be ruled out. Infections and autoimmune disease can be identified by the clinical features, course of illness, and appropriate investigations.

The aphthous ulcers in Behçet syndrome are larger and more painful than those in PFAPA, and they scar when they heal. Cyclical neutropenia generally begins within the first year of life, and the fever is due to infections that occur during the episodes of neutropenia. Cyclical neutropenia can be diagnosed by serial count of leukocytes in which the characteristic pattern of neutropenia (ANC < 500/cu mm) every 3 weeks is observed. Familial Mediterranean fever is an autosomal recessive disease with the onset of illness during childhood. It is characterized by recurrent episodes of fever lasting usually for 2 days, associated with arthritis, peritonitis, pleuritis, and rash. Most patients are of Arab, Armenian, Jewish, or Turkish descent, and a family history may be present. These children do not respond to steroid treatment and may develop amyloidosis insidiously. Hyperglobulinemia D syndrome is characterized by self-limiting episodes of fever which usually begin in infancy and might be associated with arthritis, cervical adenitis, chills, headache, macular rash, and splenomegaly. The serum IgD levels are elevated (>100 U/mL), and high levels of mevalonic acid are found in the urine during the febrile attacks.

7. *What is the treatment of PFAPA?*

Oral corticosteroids relieve symptoms of PFAPA dramatically. A single dose of prednisone (1–2 mg/kg) given at the onset of an episode can dramatically relieve the fever and other symptoms in a few hours. Corticosteroids do not decrease the number of episodes. Other proposed treatments are oral cimetidine and tonsillectomy.

23.2 Conclusion

The patient had a satisfactory response to a single dose of oral prednisone (2 mg/kg). The fever remitted in 2 h and was symptom free in 24 h. The episodes continued with the same periodicity but these episodes also responded well to a single dose of oral prednisolone. As she became older, the frequency of fever decreased and there were no episodes after the age of 8 years.

Learning Points

1. Recurrent fever without an identifiable infectious cause and with normal growth is called periodic fever, and the causes include familial Mediterranean fever, hyper-Ig D syndrome, cyclical neutropenia, and PFAPA syndrome.
2. PFAPA (periodic fever, aphthous stomatitis, pharyngitis, cervical adenitis) syndrome is an auto-inflammatory disease in which flares of inflammation cause fever and other associated symptoms.
3. PFAPA syndrome is being increasingly recognized as a relatively common cause of recurrent fever in children.
4. It is underdiagnosed due to poor awareness and lack of specific diagnostic tests.
5. Clinical criteria important for diagnosis include the following:
   (a) More than four documented stereotypical episodes of fever occurring at regular intervals of 2–8 weeks and each episode typically lasting for 2–7 days.
   (b) Pharyngitis, cervical lymphadenopathy, or aphthous ulcers during the flare.
   (c) Normal growth parameters and development with no symptoms or abnormal laboratory studies between episodes.
   (d) Resolution of symptoms (fever and pharyngitis) within hours of taking oral prednisolone (1 to 2 mg/kg).
6. Aphthous ulcers are usually on the inner lips or buccal mucosa and may be missed on physical examination, unless the child is able to point them out. Thus, careful physical examination during flares is required to identify ulcers.
7. Recognition of this clinical entity avoids unnecessary, expensive and invasive investigations.

8. PFAPA is a relatively benign and self-limited disease. The attacks become less severe, less frequent, and shorter in duration with time and cease by 10 years of age in most patients.
9. Counseling regarding the benign nature of the condition, the absence of long-term complications, and the availability of an effective treatment relieves the anxiety of the family.

Suggested Readings

Barbi E, Marzuillo P, Neri E, Naviglio S, Krauss BS. Fever in children: pearls and pitfalls. Children (Basel). 2017;4(9):81.

Vanoni F, Theodoropoulou K, Hofer M. PFAPA syndrome: a review on treatment and outcome. Pediatr Rheumatol. 2016;14(1):1–5. https://doi.org/10.1186/s12969-015-0062-4.

Wang A, Manthiram K, Dedeoglu F, Licameli GR. Periodic fever, aphthous stomatitis, pharyngitis, and adenitis (PFAPA) syndrome: a review. World J Otorhinolaryngol Head Neck Surg. 2021;7(3):166–73. https://doi.org/10.1016/j.wjorl.2021.05.004.

Suggested Readings

GPSR Compliance

The European Union's (EU) General Product Safety Regulation (GPSR) is a set of rules that requires consumer products to be safe and our obligations to ensure this.

If you have any concerns about our products, you can contact us on ProductSafety@springernature.com

In case Publisher is established outside the EU, the EU authorized representative is:

Springer Nature Customer Service Center GmbH
Europaplatz 3
69115 Heidelberg, Germany

Batch number: 10732809

Printed by Printforce, the Netherlands